THE *Skinny*
VEGAN
RECIPE BOOK

THE SKINNY VEGAN RECIPE BOOK
FRESH & DELICIOUS WHOLE FOOD PLANT BASED VEGAN RECIPES

ISBN: 978-1-912511-85-3

DISCLAIMER

CONTENTS

VEGAN SALADS

VEGAN MAIN MEALS

VEGAN DESSERTS   83

INTRODUCTION

Once your mind and your body are cared for, fuelled with the best, natural nutrients, plant-based diets can also inspire a new-found love for cooking

Changing to a plant-based diet can be advantageous for many reasons. An increase in recent years in veganism has led to a greater public focus on plant-based diets and a greater awareness of the benefits of adopting such a diet. Moving towards a plant-based diet for ecological or ethical reasons is being considered now by more people than ever; we are substantially more conscious of the environment and our impact on it, as well as more deeply appreciative of animal life.

One's physical health and wellbeing can also be greatly improved through a plant-based diet.. Concerns are often raised over the absence of meat, fish and animal products in a diet due to the nutrients and vitamins that they so greatly contribute to our bodies, however, when correctly researched, sourced and implemented, plant-based diets can match the wealth of nutrients these products offer, often providing your body with a greater range than a traditional meat-eating diet. Twists on traditional recipes for every day living can be easily adapted and enhanced with lentils and legumes, nuts and seeds and push you to explore and try new fruits and vegetables too.

Naturally nourishing your body in such a way can be incredibly effective as many of these foods boost your energy levels and fill your body with an array of antioxidants, rather than driving up cholesterol and/or blood sugar levels as many meat-heavy diets may do.

A diet heavily weighted towards vegetables, lentils, grains and fruits can dramatically aid existing health conditions and problems and help to prevent future issues. One significant health benefit of a properly maintained diet relates to controlling and maintaining a healthy weight. There is no denying that as a population, the western world now has substantial obesity problems, with the US high up the ranks, and the UK not too far behind. Obesity as a condition has an obvious array of side affects, one of the most concerning being Type II Diabetes.

The good news is that Type II Diabetes is often avoidable as it more or less stems solely from an individual being overweight. The bad and sad news is that it is not being controlled, with more and more people diagnosed with and developing the condition each year. The condition is also reversible. Lifestyles and diets need to be taken more seriously. With food and product marketing now more powerful than ever, educating and increasing awareness of food, where it comes from and how it affects our bodies is vital. Going back to basics, avoiding the additives; the microwave meals; the takeaways and gravitating towards a whole food plant-based diet can substantially improve this situation and help guide towards a healthier weight and lifestyle.

A plant-based diet involves eliminating all animal products and any by products. You may think that eating a solely plant-based diet may deprive you of essential nutrients and vitamins that our bodies need to function and thrive, but this is simply not the case. There is a wealth of foods that can be used to substitute traditional uses of fish, meat and animal produce in meals, and with these come a wide range of additional benefits, some of which you may find surprising.

A plant-based diet, which is packed with wholefoods, can keep hunger at bay. Increasing your intake of natural, unrefined grains, such as quinoa, brown rice, couscous and lentils, can actually fill you up quicker, and keep you feeling fuller for longer. This is because they are an excellent source of fibre, satisfy hormone and blood levels in our body, obtaining the nutrients and energy it requires. Only when these levels are not satisfied, such as when we eat foods high in sugar or fats, are we left feeling hungry shortly after. These grains work skilfully as a foundation for many meals filling you up quicker with the added benefit of reduced inflammation, or bloating, due to the fibre content.

Because you feel fuller consuming increased quantities of fibre you will find that naturally the portion sizes on your plate become smaller compared to a diet of refined foods. Inevitably, Many followers of a plant-based diet report weight loss as a common benefit of switching to a plant-based diet with very little effort required on their behalf to lose it.

The health benefits of increasing foods featured regularly in plant-based meals are almost endless. What we eat can affect not just our digestive system but our entire body and its functions. The increased levels of fibre associated with plant-based diets can help relieve constipation, regulate bowel movements, reduce bloating and aid conditions like Irritable Bowel Syndrome, all of which can have a substantial impact on the sufferer's daily life. Even those who do not have either diagnostic or anecdotal digestive issues report notable improvements in how they feel and look after eating: slimmer waistlines, increased energy and less stomach aches, pains and grumbles.

Obviously vegetables are a key staple to a plant-based diet and these can be used creatively in a wonder of different ways. Greens are excellent for our health and operate as an essential source of iron. Iron is largely responsible for the transportation of oxygen around our bodies, and even more essentially, is a critical component of our red blood cells through its contribution within haemoglobin. Consuming sufficient iron levels, which a plant-based diet heavily aids, helps anaemia, and generally keeps our bodies and blood cells functioning smoothly.

In addition to the vital role that iron plays in our bodies, it can also significantly improve the strength and appearance of our skin, hair and nails. Eliminating refined foods and meat from your diet can dramatically improve the appearance of skin, which can often have life changing results for sufferers of various conditions, in particular acne.

Plant-based diets are not just filled with the essential nutrients our bodies need and beneficial ones to achieve desired effects, such as clear skin or long, glossy hair, but they are also brimming with antioxidants. Antioxidants are, quite simply as the name suggests, components that prevent oxidation in the body, such as free radicals. The more antioxidants consumed, the more effective the body is at fighting off these free radicals and disabling them from developing, or growing, in the first place. This is vitally important because free radicals can harm our cells. A plant-based diet naturally rich in antioxidants helps our body prevent harm or damage to our cells, The more damage caused to our cells, the more unwell we become, either through ongoing conditions, or sometimes, through life shortening, or sadly life ending, aggressive diseases, such as cancer.

Ensuring that any diet is enriched with antioxidants is a simple, yet hugely effective, way we can try to keep our bodies as healthy as possible. Our bodies aside, plant-based diets are also great for the mind. A balanced diet, rich in fibre, nutrients, antioxidants and unrefined foods, undoubtedly boosts energy levels; one feels less sluggish and energised, their quality of sleep improves, their body, including the brain, operates more efficiently, their appearance can improve, and a healthy weight established and maintained; all of this helps towards a positive mindset and improved wellbeing. When hydrated, well rested and energised, one's approach, thoughts and actions can be very different to that of someone who is burnt out from sugar and caffeine crashes, tired & drained. In fact, when switching to a plant-based diet, a general improvement in wellbeing and mentality is often one the first things people notice, almost immediately taking its effect.

Following a whole food plant-based vegan diet is often tarnished with a brush of boring; suggesting that such a diet is restrictive, 'rabbit food' and quite frankly dull. This is far from the truth. In fact, plants, vegetables, fruits and lentils are very much what adds colour to a plate! Indeed, in the absence of fish, meat and animal produce, it is of course essential to source a balance of nutrients to optimise our bodies and its functions through alternative foods.

Gorgeous, rich oranges are now bursting into recipes through the likes of sweet potatoes and butternut squash; vibrant shades of red and plum add stunning hints to meals through the increasing use of beetroot, rhubarb and radish; and, naturally, fresh greens are brightening up meals throughout the nation as traditional greens make a resurgence and avocado and kale begin to rule the scene. Nuts, seeds, pulses and grains add fabulous texture to meals and provide a wealth of antioxidants, minerals and vitamins that, quite often are missing from the typical meat eaters diet.

Exploring a plant-based diet forces you to push outside of your day to day vegetable box, shopping list and comfort zone and opens your eyes to an array of wonderfully nutritious, delicious, vivid foods that you may have otherwise never experimented with in your cooking.

This selection of recipes offers inspiration for daily meals whilst following a traditional plant-based diet and are suitable for vegans. Once your mind and your body are cared for, fuelled with the best, natural nutrients, plant-based diets can also inspire a new-found love for cooking, as well as shopping locally and responsibly to ensure the best quality produce. Just be sure that all the ingredients you include are 100% vegan so that you can get the best out of your plant based diet.

ABOUT COOKNATION

CookNation is the leading publisher of innovative and practical recipe books for the modern, health conscious cook.CookNation titles bring together delicious, easy and practical recipes with their unique approach - easy and delicious, no-nonsense recipes - making cooking for diets and healthy eating fast, simple and fun.

With a range of #1 best-selling titles - from the innovative 'Skinny' calorie-counted series, to the 5:2 Diet Recipes collection - CookNation recipe books prove that 'Diet' can still mean 'Delicious'!

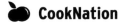 **CookNation**

Skinny
VEGAN
Breakfasts

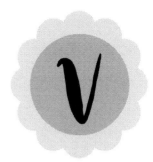

SERVES 2

TOMATOES ON TOAST

Ingredients

- 2 large plum tinned tomatoes, chopped
- ½ clove of garlic, minced
- 1 tsp tomato puree
- ½ tsp mild chilli powder
- 50g/2oz red kidney beans, cooked & drained
- 2 large sliced of wholegrain, seeded bread
- ½ tsp linseeds
- ½ tsp sunflower seeds
- A pinch of ground black pepper
- Fresh chopped basil leaf to garnish

Method

1 Place the tomatoes, garlic, tomato puree and chilli powder into a bowl and mash well until a lumpy mixture is formed.

2 Add in the kidney beans and stir well.

3 Toast the slices of bread and then spoon on top the tomato bean mixture.

4 Sprinkle over the seeds, season with a pinch of black pepper, garnish with basil and serve.

CHEF'S NOTE
For cold, winter mornings, warm the tomato and bean mixture in a pan before serving.

SIMPLY SWEET BANANA PORRIDGE

Ingredients

- 2 bananas
- ½ tbsp maple syrup
- ½ tsp desiccated coconut

- 600ml/1 pint of almond milk
- 150g/5oz organic rolled oats
- ½ tsp flaxseeds

Method

1 Place the bananas in a bowl with the maple syrup and mash them with a fork.

2 Add in the desiccated coconut, stir well and place to one side.

3 Mix the porridge oats and milk in a saucepan on a low heat.

4 Stir until the mixture begins to thicken and the oats soften.

5 Remove from the heat and add in the mashed banana mixture, stirring well.

6 Serve with a sprinkling of flaxseeds and a drizzle of any leftover maple syrup.

CHEF'S NOTE

If preferred, only mash 1 banana to stir into the porridge, slicing the other to serve on top.

CAULIFLOWER HASH BROWNS

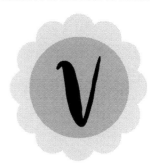

Ingredients

- ½ cauliflower head, destalked and shopped
- ½ onion, peeled & chopped
- 1 tbsp breadcrumbs
- 25g/1oz yeast
- A pinch of garlic powder

- ½ tsp fresh coriander, finely chopped
- A small pinch of turmeric
- A large pinch of sea salt and black pepper
- A splash of water
- 1 tsp sunflower oil

Method

1 Pre-heat the oven to 350F/180C /Gas 4.

2 Place the cauliflower florets in a food processor, or use a hand blender, to blend them into crumbed pieces. Do not blend to smooth or liquidise the cauliflower, just break it up to a similar size to cous cous.

3 Pour into a bowl and add in all the remaining ingredients, apart from the oil, and stir well. Use your hands to firmly knead the mixture and combine it together well.

4 From the mixture into 6 smallish, balls and use the ball of your hand to slightly flatten into thick hash browns patties.

5 Drizzle the oil over the cauliflower hash browns and place on a baking tray. Cook in the oven for 30 minutes, or until they are tender in the middle and starting to crisp on the edge.

CHEF'S NOTE
Serve with your choice of sauce, or alongside roasted tomatoes and mushrooms.

BERRY AND BANANA SPLIT YOGHURT

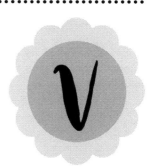

Ingredients

- 2 bananas, peeled
- 25g/1oz strawberries, quartered
- 25g/1oz raspberries, chopped
- 25g/1oz blackberries, chopped

- 2 tbsp vegan yoghurt
- 1 tbsp coconut cream
- 1 tsp maple syrup

Method

1 Using a knife, slit the bananas down the middle so they can be filled slightly but are not completely cut in half.

2 Sprinkle over the chopped berries so they sit over the bananas.

3 Mix together the vegan yoghurt and coconut cream and spoon over the bananas and berries.

4 Drizzle over the maple syrup to add some sweetness and serve.

CHEF'S NOTE
To add a crunch to this breakfast, add some crushed almonds on top.

SIMPLY SMASHED AVOCADO

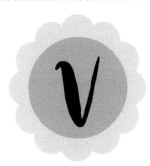

Ingredients

- 2 avocados, peeled, de-stoned & chopped
- ½ tsp olive oil
- 1 tsp freshly squeezed lime juice
- 1 large tomato, finely diced
- ½ tbsp red onion, finely diced
- 1 tsp fresh coriander, finely chopped
- A pinch of sea salt
- A large pinch of chilli flakes to garnish

Method

1 Place the avocado in a bowl with the olive oil and lime juice and mash the mixture together.

2 Add in the finely diced tomato and red onion and stir.

3 Add in the coriander, season with sea salt then combine well.

4 Garnish with a sprinkling of dried chilli flakes.

CHEF'S NOTE
Serve on toast or use as a colourful accompaniment to the cauliflower hash browns on page 14.

PEANUT BUTTER AND BLUEBERRY RICE CAKES

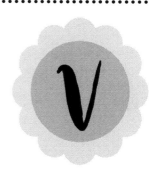

Ingredients

- 50g/2oz blueberries
- 1 tsp agave nectar
- A dash of coconut oil
- 1 tbsp vegan peanut butter

- 2 multigrain rice cakes
- A few spare whole blueberries
- 1 tsp peanuts, finely chopped
- ½ tsp poppy seeds

Method

1 Place the blueberries, agave nectar and coconut oil in a bowl and mash well until a lumpy, blueberry mixture is formed.

2 Spread the peanut butter over the rice cakes and spoon over the top of the blueberry mixture.

3 Add some whole blueberries to garnish, sprinkle over the peanuts and poppy seeds to serve.

CHEF'S NOTE
Add a spoonful of vegan yoghurt as a refreshing accompaniment.

CHEESY MUSHROOM OMELETTE

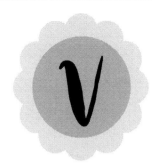

Ingredients

- 25ml/1floz soya milk
- A splash of water
- 15g/½oz chickpea flour
- A pinch of kala namak
- A pinch of garlic powder
- A large pinch of turmeric
- Sea salt & pepper to season
- 50g/2oz mushrooms, finely chopped
- 1 tbsp grated vegan cheddar cheese
- 1 tsp sunflower oil
- Freshly chopped coriander to garnish

Method

1 Simply add into a bowl the soya milk, water and flour and mix well.

2 Add in the spices and season with salt & pepper and pour the mixture into a food processor to blend it into a smooth, lump-free mixture.

3 Stir in the mushrooms and vegan cheese. Heat the sunflower oil in a small frying pan on a medium heat. Pour half of the mixture into the pan and allow it to cook for 2 – 3 minutes, or until the edges have begun to seal.

4 Carefully flip the omelette over to cook the other side for a further 2 – 3 minutes. Repeat for the second omelette and serve with a fresh coriander garnish.

CHEF'S NOTE

This is a brilliant quick and easy recipe for a staple filling breakfast; mix up the fillings as you please to create a variety of tasty omelettes.

STRAWBERRY AND APPLE SMOOTHIE

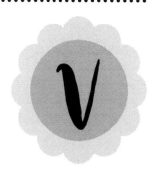

Ingredients

- 500ml/2 cups almond milk
- 1 apple
- 6 strawberries
- 1 banana, peeled
- ½ tsp fresh root ginger, grated
- 1 tsp flaxseeds
- 1 tsp hempseeds

Method

1 Peel and core the apple.

2 Peel the banana and slice the strawberries.

3 Simply add all of the ingredients into a blender, and blend until all the ingredients have smoothly combined together.

4 Serve in two glasses with ice cubes if desired.

CHEF'S NOTE

Smoothies are a great, quick and easy way to give you that breakfast energy boost you need.

SMASHED BANANA AND NUTMEG ON TOAST

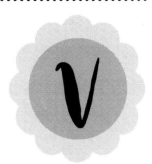

Ingredients

- 2 bananas, peeled & chopped
- 1 tsp dairy-free cream
- A small pinch of ground nutmeg

- 2 slices of granary bread
- 1 tsp flaxseeds

Method

1 Place the chopped bananas in a bowl and mash them with a fork.

2 Add in the dairy-free cream and nutmeg and mash once more, stirring the mixture well.

3 Toast the bread and then spread the banana mixture on top.

4 Sprinkle over flaxseeds to serve.

CHEF'S NOTE
Healthy breakfasts do not need to be hard work; fast but nutritious meals like this will help maintain and stabilise your energy levels to kick start your day in the most effective way.

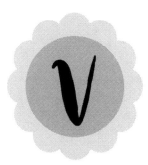

SERVES 2

SUPERCHARGED FRUITY PORRIDGE

Ingredients

- 600ml/1 pint of oat milk
- 100g/3½oz organic rolled oats
- A small pinch of salt
- 1 tbsp vegan yoghurt
- 1 tsp maple syrup
- 1 banana, peeled & chopped

- 1 kiwi, peeled & chopped
- 25g/1oz raspberries
- ½ tsp chia seeds
- ½ tsp flaxseeds
- ½ tsp poppy seeds
- ½ tsp linseeds

Method

1 Pour the oat milk into a saucepan and warm through until it begins to simmer.

2 Add in the oats and a pinch of salt and stir well. Simmer for 5 – 6 minutes, stirring frequently to ensure the mixture does not settle and stick to the bottom of the pan.

3 Once a smooth, creamy mixture has been formed, remove from the heat.

4 Spoon in the yoghurt and stir well before serving.

5 Drizzle over the maple syrup and top with the chopped fruit.

6 To serve, sprinkle over the mixed seeds.

CHEF'S NOTE
You can enrich the taste of your porridge by allowing the oats to soak overnight in the oat milk prior to cooking in the morning.

A VEGAN ENGLISH BREAKFAST

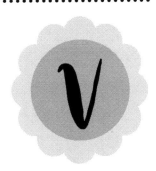

Ingredients

- 4 cauliflower hash browns (page 14)
- 4 vegan sausages
- 1 tomato, halved
- A splash of olive oil
- A pinch of sea salt
- A pinch of oregano

- 1 tsp olive oil
- ½ onion, peeled & chopped
- ½ can vegan baked beans
- 50g/2oz mushrooms, chopped
- Salt & pepper to serve

Method

1 Pre-heat the oven to 350F/180C /Gas 4. If making the cauliflower hash browns from fresh, see the Cauliflower Hash Brown recipe. If already prepared, put to one side to warm through in the oven.

2 Place the sausages on a baking tray and cook in the oven for 15 minutes. Remove the sausages from the oven and turn them over. Add the tomato halves onto the baking tray, drizzle the oil over them and sprinkle across the sea salt and oregano to season.

3 Return to the oven for a further 10 – 15 minutes, however, be sure to adjust your timings based on the recommended cooking time of the vegan sausages you purchase as this can vary.

4 5 minutes before the finish time, add in the cauliflower hash browns to warm through.

5 Meanwhile, in a pan warm the olive oil. Add in the onions and fry for 2 – 3 minutes, stirring occasionally.

6 In a small saucepan, pour in the baked beans and cook for 3 – 4 minutes, stirring regularly.

7 While these are cooking, add the mushrooms in with the onions and cook for a further 3 – 4 minutes, or until both the onion and mushrooms are tender and piping hot. Remove both pans from the heat and place to one side ready to serve.

8 Remove the sausages, tomato and hash browns from the oven and serve on a plate, alongside the onions, mushrooms and baked beans. Season with salt & pepper and serve.

ROASTED AVOCADO TOMATOES

Ingredients

- 1 large avocado, halved & de-stoned
- 2 medium tomatoes, halved
- 1 tsp olive oil
- A large pinch of sea salt & pepper
- A pinch of pine nuts
- A pinch of linseeds
- Freshly chopped parsley to garnish

Method

1 Pre-heat the oven to 350F/180C /Gas 4.

2 Place each avocado half, still with the skin on, on a baking tray and add a tomato half into the small hole where the avocado stone would have been embedded.

3 Drizzle the olive oil over the tomato and avocado and season generously with sea salt & pepper.

4 Sprinkle on top the pine nuts and linseeds and cook for 15 – 20 minutes, until the tomato is softened and beginning to crisp.

5 Simply remove from the oven and serve with fresh parsley to garnish.

CHEF'S NOTE
For a spicier version top with a pinch of chilli flakes.

WINTER BERRY COMPOTE

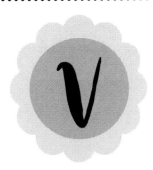

Ingredients

- 1 tsp almond butter
- 50g/2oz blackberries
- 25g/1oz blackcurrants
- 25g/1oz raspberries
- ½ tsp light brown sugar
- 150ml/5floz vegan yoghurt
- ½ tsp agave nectar
- A small handful of vegan granola
- 1 tsp chia seeds
- 1 tbsp fresh redcurrants

Method

1 Melt the almond butter in a small pan and add in the berries and sugar.

2 Simmer on a low heat for 4 – 5 minutes, stirring continuously.

3 Mash the berries with a spatula to help break them down and combine into a coulis style mixture, remove from the heat and place to one side.

4 Pour the yoghurt into a bowl and stir in the agave nectar.

5 Spoon on top of the yoghurt the winter berry coulis from the pan.

6 Sprinkle over the granola and chia seeds and top with a few redcurrants to serve.

CHEF'S NOTE
Fresh berries are bursting with whole food goodness that will boost your breakfast energy intake.

Skinny
VEGAN
Soups

SPICED BUTTERNUT SQUASH SOUP

SERVES 2

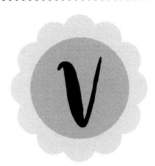

Ingredients

- 300ml/10½floz organic vegetable stock
- 3 large carrots, peeled & chopped
- ½ butternut squash, peeled & chopped
- ½ small red onion, diced
- 1 tsp fresh coriander, finely chopped
- 1 tsp red curry paste
- A large pinch of paprika
- A large pinch of sea salt
- 200ml/7floz coconut milk
- A large pinch of chilli flakes to serve

Method

1 Bring the organic vegetable stock to boil.

2 Add the carrots, butternut squash and onion to the stock and boil for 10 minutes.

3 Stir in the coriander, curry paste, paprika and salt and boil until the vegetables are tender.

4 Use a hand blender or food processor to blend until smooth.

5 Return the mixture to the pan, if removed to blend, and stir well.

6 Add in the coconut milk, continuously stirring and warm through. Serve with a pinch of chilli flakes to finish.

CHEF'S NOTE
Serve with a chunky slice of warm, homemade vegan bread.

CHUNKY ROOT VEGETABLE SOUP

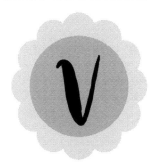

Ingredients

- 750ml/1¼ pint organic vegetable stock
- ½ onion, peeled & chopped
- 1 small potato, peeled & chopped
- 1 large carrot, peeled & chopped
- 1 turnip, peeled & chopped
- ½ celery, chopped
- A small handful of pearl barley
- 1 small bay leaf
- ½ tsp fresh basil, finely chopped
- A large splash of vegan dry white wine
- A large pinch of sea salt & pepper

Method

1 Pour the vegetable stock into a saucepan and bring to boil.

2 Add in the vegetables and stir well. Allow to boil for 5 minutes and then reduce to a medium heat and allow to simmer.

3 Add in the pearl barley, bay leaf, basil and white wine and stir well. Season with sea salt & pepper and simmer for a further 25 – 30 minutes or until the vegetables are tender.

4 Remove from the heat and serve.

CHEF'S NOTE

This soup is perfect for winter months, packed with nutrient-filled seasonal vegetables to help fight common colds.

MUSHROOM SOUP

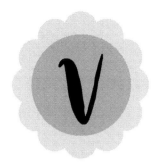

Ingredients

- 1 tbsp vegan spread
- ½ onion, peeled & chopped
- 1 small clove of garlic, minced
- ½ celery, chopped
- 250g/9oz mushrooms, chopped
- 450ml/15½floz organic vegetable stock
- 1 potato, peeled & chopped
- A large pinch of freshly chopped parsley
- A large pinch of sea salt & pepper
- Fresh parsley to garnish

Method

1 Melt the vegan spread in a saucepan on a medium heat.

2 Add in the onion, garlic and celery and cook for 5 minutes, stirring the mixture every minute or so until it has softened.

3 Add in the mushrooms and cook for a further 5 minutes, again, stirring every minute or so.

4 Pour in the vegetable stock and stir the mixture well. Add in the chopped potato and parsley and season generously with the sea salt & pepper.

5 Allow the soup to simmer for a further 25 – 30 minutes, or until the potatoes are tender.

6 Use a hand blender or food processor to blend the mixture until smooth.

7 Serve with a garnish of fresh parsley.

CHEF'S NOTE

Mushrooms are rich in the antioxidant called selenium. Antioxidants help protect against damage from aging and boost your immune system.

RAW AVOCADO, MINT AND CUCUMBER SOUP

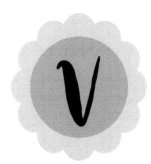

Ingredients

- 2 avocados, peeled, de-seeded & chopped
- 2 cucumbers, chopped
- 1 tsp mint, freshly chopped
- 1 tsp chives, freshly chopped
- A large pinch of freshly chopped parsley
- 2 tbsp freshly squeezed lemon juice
- 1 tbsp freshly squeezed lime juice
- 250ml/8½floz water
- A large pinch of sea salt
- Fresh parsley to season

Method

1 Simply add the avocados, cucumbers, herbs and lime and lemon juice into a food processor, or bowl if using a hand blender, and blend until a smooth mixture is created.

2 Gradually add in the water and continue to blend.

3 Season with sea salt and blend once more before serving. Garnish with fresh parsley to serve.

CHEF'S NOTE

This can be prepared a while before eating and stored in the fridge; this time allows the flavours to develop further.

BROCCOLI AND BASIL SOUP

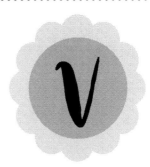

Ingredients

- 450ml/15½floz organic vegetable stock
- 1 large broccoli head, destalked & chopped
- 25g / 1oz fresh basil leaves, finely chopped
- ¼ onion, peeled & chopped

- 1 clove of garlic, minced
- 1 tsp oregano, finely chopped
- A pinch of sea salt & pepper
- 1 tbsp coconut cream
- Fresh basil leaves to garnish

Method

1 Bring the vegetable stock to boil and add in the broccoli.

2 Simmer for 5 minutes on a medium heat. Add in the basil leaves, onion, garlic and oregano and mix well.

3 Season with salt & pepper. Allow the mixture to simmer for a further 15 minutes, or until the broccoli and basil is delicately tender.

4 Pour the mixture into a food processor, or blend with a hand blender, until a smooth mixture is created. Pour into a bowl and gently drizzle in a spoonful of coconut cream to serve.

5 Garnish with fresh basil.

CHEF'S NOTE
Broccoli is a great source of vitamins K and C, a good source of folate (folic acid).

CREAMY BEETROOT SOUP

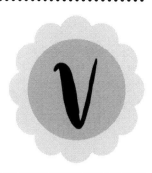

Ingredients

- 450ml/15½floz vegetable stock
- 400g/14oz beetroot, chopped
- 50g/2oz tinned chopped tomatoes
- ½ red onion, peeled & finely chopped
- 1 leek, finely chopped
- 2 cloves of garlic, minced

- 1 tsp freshly squeezed lemon juice
- 1 tsp dairy-free horseradish
- A large pinch of sea salt & pepper
- 1 tbsp vegan yoghurt
- Fresh chopped thyme leaves to garnish

Method

1 Bring the vegetable stock to boil. Add in the beetroot, tomatoes, onion and leek and boil for 2 – 3 minutes. Reduce the heat and allow the mixture to simmer.

2 Add in the garlic, lemon juice and horseradish and season with salt & pepper.

3 Stir well and gently simmer for 30 – 35 minutes or until the beetroot, onion and leeks are tender.

4 Then, either pour the mixture into a food processor or use a hand blender to blend it into a smooth, lump-free mixture, ready to serve.

5 Drizzle in some of the yoghurt and garnish with fresh thyme to serve.

CHEF'S NOTE

This soup is a gorgeously rich colour and packed with nutrients; beetroot has also been linked with reducing high bloody pressure.

PARSNIP, AGAVE AND GARLIC SOUP

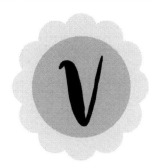

Ingredients

- 450ml/15½floz vegetable stock
- 375g/13oz parsnips, peeled & chopped
- ½ onion, peeled & finely chopped
- ½ leek, finely chopped
- ½ tbsp agave nectar
- ½ tsp freshly squeezed lemon juice

- 1 tsp unrefined brown sugar
- A pinch of ground black pepper
- ½ tsp fresh parsley, finely chopped
- 60ml/2floz coconut cream
- Fresh chopped parsley to garnish

Method

1 Bring the vegetable stock to boil.

2 Add in the parsnips, onion and celery and simmer for 10 minutes. Then, add in the agave, lemon juice, sugar, pepper and parsley, mix well and allow the mixture to simmer for a further 10 – 12 minutes, or until the parsnips are tender.

3 Stir in the coconut cream and allow it to warm through. Pour the mixture into a food processor, or use a hand blender, and blend until a smooth mixture is created.

4 Garnish with fresh parsley to serve.

CHEF'S NOTE
Parsnips are a good source of vitamin C, folate and manganese.

SERVES 2

TOFU NOODLE SOUP

Ingredients

- 600ml/1 pint of vegetable stock
- ½ onion, peeled & chopped
- 1 small carrot, chunkily grated
- ¼ leek, finely chopped
- ½ clove of garlic, minced

- A pinch of sea salt & pepper
- 1 tsp coconut oil
- 50g/2oz tofu, diced
- 50g/2oz whole wheat udon noodles
- Fresh parsley to season

Method

1 Bring the vegetable stock to boil and add in the onion, carrot, leek and garlic. Let the mixture simmer for 10 minutes. Heat the coconut oil in a pan on a medium heat.

2 Add the tofu to the pan, having gently pressed it to remove excess moisture. Cook for 5 minutes, turning the tofu half way through, or until the tofu is a light golden colour.

3 Once cooked, place the tofu in the saucepan with the simmering vegetables, then add in the udon noodles.

4 Simmer for a further few minutes, or until the noodles are cooked through. Serve the soup as it is and garnish with a pinch of fresh parsley leaf.

CHEF'S NOTE

Using whole wheat udon noodles ensures the most nutritional benefits, including the bran and the germ's vitamin E, major B vitamins, antioxidants, appetite-squashing fibre, protein and healthy fats.

FIERY TOMATO AND LENTIL SOUP

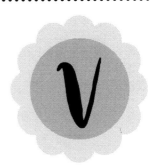

Ingredients

- 450ml/15½floz vegetable stock
- 200g/7oz tinned plum tomatoes, chopped
- ½ red onion, finely chopped
- 1 celery stick, finely chopped
- 1 carrot, peeled & chopped

- 1 small potato, peeled & diced
- 25g/1oz red lentils
- 25g/1oz yellow split peas
- 15g/½oz green lentils
- Pinch of fresh root ginger, grated
- 1 clove of garlic, minced

- ½ red chilli, de-seeded & finely sliced
- 1 tsp ground paprika
- 1 tbsp fresh coriander, finely chopped
- Sea salt and black pepper
  Fresh parsley to garnish

Method

1 Bring the vegetable stock to boil and add in the chopped plum tomatoes along with the juices from the tin.

2 Add in the onion, celery, carrot and potato and simmer for 5 minutes.

3 Add in the lentils, ginger, garlic, chilli, paprika and coriander and then season with salt & pepper.

4 Stir the mixture well and allow to simmer for 20 – 25 minutes so that the vegetables are tender.

5 Serve the soup as it is and garnish with fresh chopped parsley.

CHEF'S NOTE
Lentils are a great source of folate and magnesium, which are big contributors to heart health.

SERVES 2

SPICED SWEET POTATO AND CARROT SOUP

Ingredients

- 450ml/15½floz vegetable stock
- 200g/7oz sweet potatoes, peeled & chopped
- 100g/3½oz carrot, peeled & chopped
- 75g/3oz butternut squash, chopped
- ½ onion, peeled & chopped
- ½ tsp nutmeg

- ½ tsp cumin
- A pinch of ground cloves
- 100ml/3½floz coconut milk
- A pinch brown sugar
- 1 tbsp vegan yoghurt
- 1 tsp sunflower seeds

Method

1 Bring the vegetable stock to boil. Add in the sweet potatoes, carrots, butternut squash and onion and boil for 10 minutes.

2 Add in the spices and allow the soup to simmer for a further 15 minutes, or until the vegetables are tender.

3 Keeping on a low heat, stir in the coconut milk and a pinch of brown sugar.

4 Use a hand blender or food processor to blend until a smooth, lump-free texture. To serve, drizzle on top some yoghurt, creating a circular pattern of your choice and top with sunflower seeds.

CHEF'S NOTE

Sweet potatoes are a rich source of fibre and are bursting with goodness including iron, calcium, selenium, plus they're a good source of most of our B vitamins and vitamin C.

LEEK AND SWEETCORN SOUP

SERVES 2

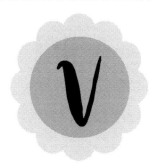

Ingredients

- 1 tsp dairy-free spread
- 1 leek, chopped
- 1 celery stick, chopped
- ½ spring onion, chopped
- 1 clove of garlic, minced
- Sea salt & pepper.
- 600ml/1 pint vegetable stock

- 1 small potato, peeled & chopped
- A large handful of frozen sweetcorn
- 1 tbsp fresh tarragon, finely chopped
- 2 tbsp dry white wine
- A pinch of ground black pepper
- 1 tbsp dairy-free cream to serve

Method

1 Heat the spread in the pan and sauté the leek, celery, spring onion and garlic on a medium heat, seasoning generous with sea salt & pepper.

2 Cook for a few minutes, until the vegetables begin to soften.

3 Bring the vegetable stock to boil and add in the potato, along with the leek mixture from the pan.

4 Add in the sweetcorn, tarragon and white wine and stir well. Allow to simmer for 30 – 35 minutes or until the vegetables are tender.

5 Serve with a pinch of black pepper and a drizzle of cream on top.

CHEF'S NOTE
Double check the wine is vegan, many wines are clarified using animal products.

MOROCCAN STYLE SOUP

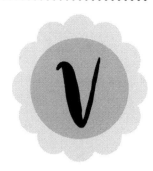

Ingredients

- 1 tsp olive oil
- ½ onion, peeled & chopped
- 1 celery stick, chopped
- 1 tsp fresh root ginger, grated
- 400g/14oz tinned tomatoes
- 25g/1oz red lentils
- 25g/1oz green lentils

- 450ml/15½floz vegetable stock
- 25g/1oz chickpeas, cooked & drained
- 1 tsp ground turmeric
- 1 tsp ground cinnamon
- 1 tsp paprika

- ½ tsp saffron
- ½ tbsp fresh coriander, finely chopped
- ½ tbsp fresh parsley, finely chopped
- Fresh coriander to garnish

Method

1 Heat the oil in the pan and sauté the onion and celery for 2 – 3 minutes.

2 Add in the ginger and cook for a further 2 – 3 minutes until they begin to soften. Remove from the heat and place to one side.

3 In a saucepan, add the tinned tomatoes and vegetable stock and bring to a boil.

4 Reduce the heat and allow the mixture to simmer. Add in the chickpeas, lentils, herbs and spices and simmer for 30 – 35 minutes.

5 Remove from the heat and serve with a coriander garnish.

CHEF'S NOTE
The longer you leave this to simmer, the more the flavours develop.

SPLIT GREEN PEA SOUP

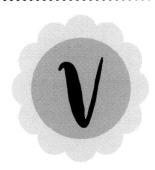

Ingredients

- 1 tsp olive oil
- ½ onion, peeled & chopped
- ½ celery stick, chopped
- 1 clove of garlic, minced
- 1 carrot, peeled & chopped
- 450ml/15½floz vegetable stock
- 125g/4oz frozen peas

- 200g/7oz split green peas
- 1 small bay leaf
- 1 tsp fresh thyme, finely chopped
- ½ tsp mint, dried
- Sea salt & pepper to season
- Fresh mint leaves to garnish

Method

1 Heat the oil in the pan and sauté the onion, celery, garlic and carrot for 3 – 4 minutes, until they begin to soften. Remove from the heat and place to one side.

2 Bring the vegetable stock to boil and add in the contents from the pan, along with the frozen peas and split green peas.

3 Allow to simmer for 5 minutes. Then, add in the bay leaf, thyme and mint and season generously with sea salt & pepper. Simmer for a further 30 – 35 minutes.

4 Once the vegetables are tender, remove from the heat and either serve as it is, or used a hand blender to smooth the mixture, if preferred. Garnish with a fresh mint leaf to serve.

CHEF'S NOTE
Peas are protein rich and a good source of fibre.

HEALING LEMON TOFU SOUP

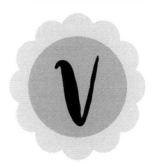

Ingredients

- 75g/3oz firm tofu
- 600ml/1 pint of water
- ½ onion, peeled & chopped
- ½ celery stick, chopped
- 1 ½ cloves of garlic, minced
- 1 tbsp freshly squeezed lemon juice
- ½ tsp fresh lemon zest, grated

- A pinch of fresh dill, finely chopped
- A large pinch of fresh oregano, finely chopped
- 2 bay leaves
- A large pinch of black pepper
- 50g/2oz pearl barley
- A small pinch of sesame seeds to serve

Method

1 Gently press the firm tofu with a kitchen towel to remove any excess water before cooking.

2 Place a saucepan on a medium heat and bring the water to boil. Add in the onion, celery, garlic and tofu and simmer for 5 minutes.

3 Reduce to a low heat and add in the lemon juice, zest and herbs, and season generously with black pepper. Allow the soup to simmer for a further 5 minutes.

4 Then, add in the pearl barley and simmer for another 20 – 25 minutes. You can keep on a low heat and cook for longer if desired.

5 Remove from the heat and serve with a sprinkling of sesame seeds.

CHEF'S NOTE

Sesame seeds are an excellent source of copper and a very good source of manganese.

Skinny
VEGAN
Salads

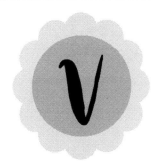

SERVES 2

CHILLI AND CUCUMBER SALAD

Ingredients

- 1 tbsp olive oil
- ½ tsp lime juice, freshly squeezed
- Small pinch of freshly chopped mint
- 1 large handful of iceberg lettuce, chopped
- A small, loose handful of fresh basil leaves
- ½ cucumber, cut into ribbons or thin strips
- ½ fresh red chilli, de-seeded & finely sliced
- A pinch of chill flakes
- 1 tsp sesame seeds

Method

1 Mix the oil, lime juice and mint together to create the dressing and place to one side.

2 Toss the lettuce and basil leaves together and put on plates ready to serve as the salad base.

3 Arrange the cucumber ribbons on top of the salad.

4 Scatter over the sliced red chilli and drizzle the salad in the salad dressing.

5 Sprinkle over the salad the chilli flakes and sesame seeds and serve.

CHEF'S NOTE
Add a small portion of brown rice or quinoa for an extra energy boosting warm salad.

MANGO AND HALLOUMI SALAD

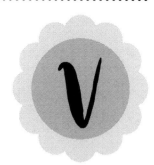

Ingredients

- 1 tbsp olive oil
- ½ tsp lime juice, freshly squeezed
- Sea salt & pepper
- 2 large handfuls of baby leaf salad leaves
- 1 small, ripe mango, peeled & chopped
- ½ avocado, peeled, de-seeded & chopped
- 200g/7oz vegan halloumi, sliced
- 1 tsp pine nuts
- 1 tsp pumpkin seeds
- ½ tsp sesame seeds

Method

1 Mix the olive oil and the lime juice together and season with the sea salt & pepper. Place to one side to use as the salad dressing.

2 Toss the salad leaves, mango and avocado in a bowl ready to serve.

3 Place a frying pan on a medium heat and allow the pan to warm, but not get too hot. Do not use any oil or butter alternative, but dry cook the halloumi.

4 Cook for 2 – 3 minutes, or until the halloumi is starting to 'sweat' and then turn the halloumi over to cook the other side.

5 Once cooked, remove from the pan and place on top of the salad. Drizzle over the dressing and sprinkle across the pine nuts, sunflower and sesame seeds to serve.

CHEF'S NOTE
Mango works brilliantly in salads, adding a great, but subtle, flavour and texture and is fantastic for giving your skin a clear, healthy glow.

ROASTED BEETROOT & SWEET POTATO SALAD

SERVES 2

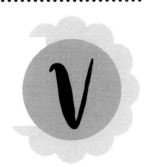

Ingredients

- 100g/3½oz sweet potatoes, peeled & chopped
- 1 beetroot, peeled & chopped
- 1 tsp soybean oil
- A large pinch of sea salt
- ½ tsp olive oil
- A splash of freshly squeezed lime juice
- Small pinch of sea salt & pepper
- 2 large handfuls of fresh baby leaf salad
- 1 tsp pumpkin seeds
- 1 tsp chia seeds
- 1 tsp pine nuts

Method

1 Pre-heat the oven to 350F/180C /Gas 4.

2 Toss the chopped sweet potatoes and beetroot in the soybean oil and season well with sea salt.

3 Place in the oven and roast for 40 – 45 minutes, or until the vegetables are tender.

4 Mix the olive oil, lime juice and salt & pepper in together to create a light dressing and place to one side ready to serve.

5 Place the salad leaves in a bowl or plate to serve and lightly toss in some of the salad dressing.

6 Once cooked, add on top the beetroot and sweet potatoes and use any additional dressing leftover that you wish to.

7 Sprinkle over the seeds and nuts and serve.

CHEF'S NOTE
A wonderful warm and filling salad full of gorgeous colours that can easily be kept for lunch the following day.

WARM MEDITERRANEAN SALAD

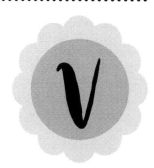

Ingredients

- ½ red onion, peeled & chopped
- ½ red pepper, de-seeded & chopped
- ½ yellow pepper, de-seeded & chopped
- ¼ courgette, chopped
- 1 large tomato, chopped
- 50g/2oz olives, pitted

- 1 tbsp olive oil
- ½ tsp freshly squeezed lemon juice
- ½ clove of garlic, peeled & finely chopped
- A large pinch of sea salt & pepper
- Fresh coriander to serve

Method

1 Pre-heat the oven to 350F/180C /Gas 4.

2 Add all the vegetables into a roasting dish and drizzle over the oil and lemon juice.

3 Add in the garlic and season well with a generous pinch of salt & pepper.

4 Toss the vegetables in the oil and seasoning until well covered.

5 Place in the oven for 30 – 35 minutes, or until the vegetables are tender. Once cooked, remove from the oven.

6 Garnish with some fresh coriander to serve.

CHEF'S NOTE
Serve with a side of quinoa, couscous or crushed potatoes for a hearty, vibrant dinner.

ROASTED AUBERGINE AND TOMATO SALAD

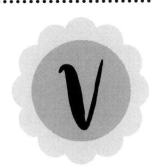

Ingredients

- ½ red onion, peeled & chopped
- 1 aubergine, chopped lengthways
- 1 courgette, chopped lengthways
- 75g/3oz cherry tomatoes, halved
- 1 tsp olive oil
- ½ clove of garlic, minced

- ½ tsp freshly squeezed lime juice
- ½ tsp freshly squeezed lemon juice
- A large pinch of sea salt & pepper
- 100g/3½oz kidney beans
- A splash of balsamic vinegar
- 1 tsp pumpkin seeds

Method

1 Pre-heat the oven to 350F/180C /Gas 4.

2 Toss the onion, aubergine, courgette and tomatoes in the olive oil, garlic, lime and lemon juice and place on a baking tray.

3 Season well with sea salt & pepper and place in the oven to roast for 20 – 25 minutes or until tender.

4 Add the kidney beans to a small pan of water and simmer on a medium heat until warmed through.

5 Once cooked, remove the vegetables from the oven and drain the kidney beans.

6 Mix them all together, stirring well and add a splash of balsamic vinegar and top with pumpkin seeds to serve.

CHEF'S NOTE
Add variety to this warm salad by adding in some tofu or vegan halloumi.

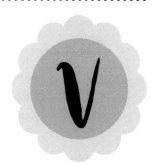

SERVES 2

LEMON AND FENNEL TOFU SALAD

Ingredients

- 1 tbsp olive oil
- ½ tsp freshly squeezed lemon juice
- A pinch of sea salt & pepper
- 50g/2oz flageolet beans
- 1 tsp olive oil
- 50g/2oz firm tofu, chopped
- The zest of ½ lemon
- 1 small fennel bulb, finely chopped
- ½ onion, peeled and roughly chopped
- 2 large handfuls of fresh rocket leaves
- 1 tsp linseeds
- 1 tsp pine nuts

Method

1 Mix the olive oil and lemon juice together and season with sea salt & pepper to make a light dressing, place to one side ready to serve.

2 Add the flageolet beans to a small pan of water and simmer until warmed through. Remove from the heat, drain and place to one side.

3 Heat the olive oil in a pan on a medium heat and add the tofu to the pan, having gently pressed it to remove excess moisture. Cook for 5 minutes, turning the tofu half way through, or until the tofu is a light golden colour.

4 Place the drained flageolet beans and tofu into a bowl and add in the lemon zest, fennel, raw onion and rocket leaves and toss well. Add in the linseeds and pine nuts and drizzle over the salad dressing. Toss well again and serve.

CHEF'S NOTE
To get your taste buds tingling, add in some fresh red chilli when cooking the tofu to give the salad a powerful kick.

47

THAI-INSPIRED APPLE AND CABBAGE SALAD

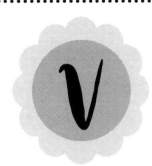

Ingredients

- ½ tbsp light soy sauce
- ½ clove of garlic, minced
- ½ green chilli, de-seeded & finely chopped
- 1 tsp freshly squeezed lime juice
- 1 tsp unrefined, brown sugar
- 1 gala apple, cored and sliced

- 1 large carrot, grated
- ½ white cabbage, grated
- ½ cucumber, finely sliced lengthways
- 1 tbsp sunflower seeds
- 1 tbsp peanuts
- A large pinch of sesame seeds

Method

1 Mix the soy sauce, garlic, chilli, lime juice and sugar together, stirring well to create a dressing for the salad and place to one side.

2 Add the apple, carrot, cabbage and cucumber into a bowl and toss together.

3 Drizzle over the dressing and sprinkle in the seeds and peanuts and toss well before serving.

CHEF'S NOTE

Add even more texture to this salad by including some halloumi and turn it into a filling dinner.

AVOCADO, LIME AND BEETROOT SALAD

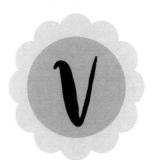

Ingredients

- 1 tbsp olive oil
- 1 tsp freshly squeezed lime juice
- ½ tsp freshly chopped coriander
- 100g/3½oz black beans
- 2 large handfuls of fresh baby leaf salad
- ¼ cucumber, finely chopped
- zest of ½ lime, finely grated
- 1 avocado, peeled, de-seeded & chopped
- 1 cooked beetroot, finely diced
- Fresh coriander to garnish

Method

1 Mix together the oil, lime juice and coriander to create a light dressing and place to one side ready to serve.

2 Add the black beans to a pan of water and simmer until warmed through. Remove from the heat, drain and place to one side.

3 Mix in a bowl the salad leaves, cucumber, lime zest, avocado and beetroot and toss well.

4 Drizzle over the prepared salad dressing and add a coriander leaf to garnish.

CHEF'S NOTE

For a warming alternative, roast the beetroot and serve straight from the oven with a brown rice base.

SUPER GREEN BEAN AND GARLIC SALAD

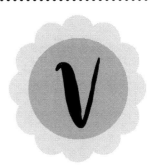

Ingredients

- ½ tbsp olive oil
- ½ clove of garlic, minced
- ½ tsp freshly chopped coriander
- A handful of new potatoes, halved
- ½ courgette, finely diced
- 75g/3oz fresh green beans, chopped
- 50g/2oz fresh mangetout
- 50g/2oz tinned broad beans
- 1 tsp sunflower seeds
- 1 tsp cashew nuts, chopped

Method

1 Mix the oil, garlic and coriander together to create a light garlic dressing and place to one side ready to serve.

2 Add the new potatoes into a pan of water, bring to boil and cook until tender.

3 Meanwhile gently fry the green beans, courgette, mangetout & broad beans in a little olive oil for a few minutes.

4 Drain the potatoes and combined with the sautéed vegetables.

5 Drizzle over the prepared dressing and add in the sunflower seeds & chopped cashew nuts.

6 Toss well and serve.

CHEF'S NOTE
Fully of antioxidants and iron, this salad is a brilliant immune system boosting meal.

ORANGE AND HARISSA WARM SALAD

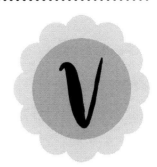

Ingredients

- 300ml/10½floz vegetable stock
- 100g/3½oz brown rice
- ½ tbsp freshly squeezed lemon juice
- 1 tbsp agave nectar
- 1 tsp harissa paste
- 1 tbsp flaxseed oil
- A handful of finely chopped red onion

- ½ spring onion, finely chopped
- 1 tbsp fresh parsley, finely chopped
- 1 large orange, peeled and segmented
- 1 tbsp chia seeds
- 1 tsp sesame seeds
- A large pinch of alfalfa sprouts

Method

1 Bring the vegetable stock to boil and add in the rice. Simmer for 15-20 minutes or until cooked through.

2 Drain the rice and place in a bowl.

3 Add the lemon juice, agave nectar, harissa paste and olive oil to the rice and stir well.

4 Mix in the red onion, spring onion and parsley. Then, add in the orange segments, followed by the seeds and stir well before serving.

5 Garnish with a large pinch of sprouts to serve.

CHEF'S NOTE
Using stock to cook grains and lentils through adds a greater flavour.

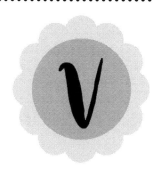

SUPER SIMPLE BRITISH GARDEN SALAD

SERVES 2

Ingredients

- 1 tbsp olive oil
- ½ tsp freshly squeezed lemon juice
- A small pinch of sea salt & pepper
- ¼ iceberg lettuce, chopped
- ¼ cucumber, chopped
- A large handful of cherry tomatoes, halved
- 1 radish, finely sliced
- 1 spring onion, finely sliced

Method

1 Mix the olive oil with the lemon juice, season with salt & pepper, and place to one side to use as the dressing later on.

2 Simply toss the lettuce, cucumber, tomatoes, radish and onion together in a bowl.

3 Drizzle over some of the prepared salad dressing and serve.

CHEF'S NOTE
Sprinkle in a mixture of nuts and seeds of your choice to add texture, colour and extra nutrients to this super simple salad.

AGAVE AND MUSTARD SALAD

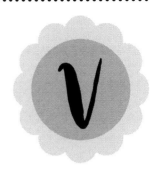

Ingredients

- 1 tbsp olive oil
- 1 tsp wholegrain vegan mustard
- 1 tsp agave nectar
- A dash of freshly squeezed lemon juice
- 2 large handfuls of fresh rocket leaves
- 1 handful of fresh baby leaf salad leaves
- ¼ cucumber, chopped
- ½ avocado, peeled, de-stoned & chopped
- 1 tsp chia seeds
- 1 tsp sunflower seeds

Method

1 Mix together the olive oil, wholegrain mustard, agave and lemon juice and place to one side to use as the dressing later.

2 Simply toss the salad leaves, cucumber, avocado and seeds together.

3 Drizzle over some of the salad dressing and serve.

CHEF'S NOTE

The agave offsets the sharpness of the mustard providing a delicious homemade dressing.

BEETROOT AND APPLE SALAD

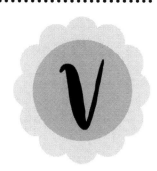

Ingredients

- 200g/7oz cooked beetroot, diced
- 1 gala apple, cored & diced
- Handful of cherry tomatoes, finely chopped
- ½ tsp fresh mint, finely chopped
- ½ tsp fresh coriander, finely chopped
- ½ tsp flaxseed oil
- A splash of freshly squeezed lemon juice
- A splash of balsamic vinegar
- 1 tsp chia seeds
- 1 tsp sunflower seeds
- 1 tsp pomegranate seeds

Method

1 Add the cooked beetroot, apple and tomatoes into a bowl and toss well together.

2 Mix in the mint and coriander and drizzle over the oil and lemon juice.

3 Add a splash of balsamic vinegar and sprinkle in the seeds. Toss the salad well and serve.

CHEF'S NOTE
Beetroots are an excellent source of folic acid and a very good source of fibre, manganese and potassium.

SPICY SALSA-STYLE SALAD

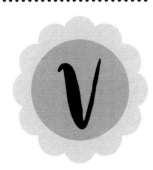

Ingredients

- 1 tsp olive oil
- ½ tsp freshly squeezed lime juice
- 1 tbsp fresh coriander, finely chopped
- A pinch of garlic powder
- 150g/5oz cherry tomatoes, finely chopped
- ½ red pepper, de-seeded & finely diced
- ¼ yellow pepper, de-seeded & finely diced
- ¼ red onion, peeled & finely diced
- 4 sundried tomatoes, chopped
- ½ small green chilli, de-seeded & finely sliced
- ½ tsp paprika
- 1 tsp pine nuts

Method

1 Place the olive oil, lime juice, coriander and garlic into a bowl and mix well to create a light salad dressing ready to serve and put to one side.

2 Simply add the tomatoes, peppers, onion, sundried tomatoes, chilli and paprika into another bowl and toss well together.

3 Drizzle over the prepared dressing and pine nuts and serve.

CHEF'S NOTE
Serve on a fresh bed of salad or a toasted flatbread.

SPINACH AND GREEN BEAN SALAD

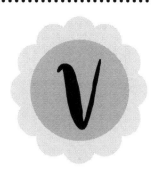

Ingredients

- 100g/3½oz green beans, sliced lengthways
- 1 tsp olive oil
- A splash of freshly squeezed lemon juice
- A pinch of garlic powder
- ½ tsp ground cumin

- A pinch of chilli powder
- A pinch of freshly chopped mint
- 150g/5oz spinach
- A handful of fresh basil leaves
- A handful of fresh baby leaf salad leaves

- 1 spring onion, finely chopped
- 1 tsp peanuts, chopped
- 1 tsp toasted almonds, chopped
- Lemon zest to serve

Method

1 Bring a saucepan of water to boil and add in the green beans. Simmer for a few minutes until slightly tender but still firm.

2 Meanwhile, mix the olive oil, lemon juice, garlic, cumin, chilli powder and mint together in a bowl to prepare a salad dressing and place to one side ready to serve.

3 Drain the beans and combine with the spinach.

4 Sprinkle over the spring onion, peanuts and toasted almonds. Drizzle over the salad dressing and garnish with some grated lemon zest to serve.

CHEF'S NOTE
Spinach is a fantastic source of iron and can be easily added to almost any salad for a nutrient-filled energy boost.

ASPARAGUS, PISTACHIO AND SUNFLOWER SEED SALAD

Ingredients

- 200g/7oz asparagus
- 1 tbsp pistachio nuts, shelled & chopped
- 2 tsp sunflower oil
- A pinch of sea salt
- ½ tsp freshly squeezed lemon juice
- 1 tsp coconut cream

- ½ tsp agave nectar
- 1 tsp fresh thyme, finely chopped
- 2 large handfuls of fresh rocket leaves
- 2 tsp sunflower seeds
- Fresh thyme leaves to garnish

Method

1 Pre-heat the oven to 400F/200C /Gas 6.

2 Place the asparagus in a roasting dish along with the pistachio nuts and drizzle over 1 tsp of the sunflower oil.

3 Turn the asparagus and nuts so they are evenly coated in oil and season with sea salt. Roast in the oven for 15 minutes, or until the asparagus is tender.

4 Meanwhile, mix in a bowl the remaining sunflower oil, the lemon juice, coconut cream, agave nectar and fresh thyme. Stir well and place to one side ready to serve.

5 Once cooked, remove the asparagus from the oven and serve on top of a bed of rocket leaves.

6 Drizzle over the dressing and top with the roasted pistachio nuts from the oven and the sunflower seeds. Garnish with a fresh thyme leaf and serve.

CHEF'S NOTE

Nuts contain a fabulous range of nutrients and antioxidants as well as being packed with protein.

SPICY BEAN SALAD

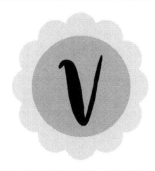

Ingredients

- 50g / 2oz butter beans, cooked & drained
- 50g / 2oz kidney beans, cooked & drained
- 50g / 2oz chickpeas, cooked & drained
- 1 tbsp green split peas, cooked & drained
- ½ tsp olive oil
- 200g/7oz chopped tomatoes

- 1 tsp tomato puree
- 1 tsp ground paprika
- 1 tsp chilli powder
- ¼ red chilli, de-seeded & finely sliced
- A pinch of garlic powder

Method

1 Toss the cooked beans, chickpeas and split peas together in a bowl.

2 Heat the olive oil in a frying pan. Add to the pan the chopped tomatoes and allow to simmer for 2 minutes. Add in the tomato puree paprika, chilli powder, red chilli and garlic and allow to simmer on a low heat for a further 5 minutes, stirring occasionally, until a thick mixture is created. If still watery, continue to simmer for a few more minutes.

3 Remove from the heat and spoon the sauce into the bowl of beans and mix well, read to serve.

CHEF'S NOTE
Serve on a large, fresh bed of salad leaves of your choice.

MANGO AND ASPARAGUS SALAD

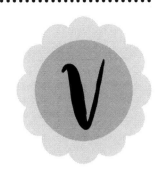

Ingredients

- 200g / 7oz asparagus
- 1 tsp olive oil
- A pinch of sea salt
- 1 tsp avocado oil
- ½ tsp freshly squeezed lime juice
- A pinch of ground black pepper
- A large handful of spinach

- 100g / 3½oz mango, peeled & chopped
- ½ cucumber, diced
- ½ avocado, peeled, de-stoned & diced
- 1 tsp pine nuts
- 1 tsp sesame seeds
- 1 tsp chia seeds

Method

1 Pre-heat the oven to 400F/200C /Gas 6.

2 Drizzle the asparagus in the olive oil and season with salt. Roast for 15 minutes, or until the asparagus is tender.

3 Bring a pan of water to boil while you prepare a simple salad dressing: mix the avocado oil, lime juice and black pepper in a small bowl and place to one side, ready to serve.

4 Add the spinach into the pan of boiling water and simmer for until the spinach begins to wilt.

5 Once cooked, remove the asparagus from the oven, and drain the spinach.

6 Place in a bowl with the mango, cucumber and avocado. Toss the ingredients together well. Add in the nuts and seeds and toss once more.

7 Drizzle over the prepared salad dressing and serve.

CHEF'S NOTE
Serve on a fresh bed of rocket leaves, or with brown rice to keep you feeling even fuller for longer.

SPRING ONION AND RED CHILLI SALAD

Ingredients

- 100g / 3½oz brown rice
- 1 tsp flaxseed oil
- 3 spring onions, finely chopped
- 1 red chilli, de-seeded & finely sliced
- 1 clove of garlic, minced
- A pinch of fresh root ginger, grated
- 2 tsp fresh lemongrass, finely chopped

- 50ml / 2floz vegetable stock
- 1 tsp freshly squeezed lime juice
- A pinch of lime zest, grated
- 2 tsp soy sauce
- ½ cucumber shredded
- 1 tsp sesame seeds

Method

1 Bring a pan of water to boil and cook the rice until the rice is tender.

2 Meanwhile, warm the oil in a frying pan and on a low heat cook the spring onions, chilli, garlic, ginger and lemongrass and cook for 2 – 3 minutes, stirring frequently.

3 Add in the vegetable stock, lime juice, lime zest and soy sauce and stir well. Allow the mixture to simmer for a further 5 minutes, or until the ingredients are tender.

4 Once cooked, drain the rice and return it to the saucepan.

5 Spoon in the spring onion and red chilli mixture from the pan and mix well with the rice.

6 Add in the shredded cucumber and give one final mix before serving.

7 Sprinkle on top sesame seeds and serve.

CHEF'S NOTE

The health benefits of brown rice are due to it being a whole grain. The fibre helps lower cholesterol, moves waste through the digestive tract, promotes fullness, and helps prevent the formation of blood clots.

OLIVE AND ORANGE SALAD

Ingredients

- 1 tsp olive oil
- A splash of freshly squeezed lemon juice
- A pinch of ground black pepper
- 2 oranges, peeled and segmented
- A hand of mixed olives, chopped
- ½ red onion, peeled & finely sliced
- ½ green chilli, de-seeded & finely sliced
- ½ fennel bulb, finely sliced
- ½ clove of garlic, finely sliced
- ½ tsp fresh parsley, finely chopped
- 1 tsp pine nuts
- A pinch of fresh parsley leaf to garnish

Method

1 Mix the olive oil, lemon juice and black pepper together in a small bowl and place to one side, ready to serve as a light, simple dressing.

2 Simply add the oranges, olives, onion and chilli in a bowl and toss together.

3 Drizzle over the prepared dressing and stir well.

4 Add in the chilli, fennel, garlic and parsley and mix well. Spoon the salad onto a plate to serve and top with a sprinkling of pine nuts.

5 Garnish with a fresh parsley leaf to serve.

CHEF'S NOTE
This is a perfect raw salad for summer, but also makes an excellent light snack for dinner or cocktail parties.

Skinny
VEGAN
Main Meals

FREEKEH AND THYME STUFFED TOMATOES

SERVES 2

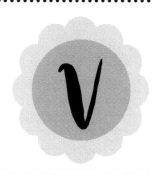

Ingredients

- 6 large tomatoes, halved
- 1 tbsp hempseed oil
- ½ tsp brown sugar
- 175ml/6floz water
- 50g/2oz freekeh
- 1 clove of garlic, minced
- ½ small red onion, peeled & finely chopped
- 1 tsp paprika, ground
- ½ tsp mild chilli powder
- 1 tsp fresh thyme, finely chopped
- A splash of olive oil
- Sea salt & pepper to season
- 2 large handfuls of fresh rocket leaves
- 1 tsp pine nuts

Method

1 Pre-heat the oven to 350F/180C /Gas 4.

2 Hollow out the tomatoes and drizzle over the hempseed oil so the tomatoes are evenly covered.

3 Sprinkle in the brown sugar to sweeten them slightly before roasting. Place the tomatoes in a roasting dish and cook for 30 – 35 minutes or until they begin to shrivel.

4 Bring the water to boil. Rinse the freekeh first and then add it in to the water to simmer for 20 – 25 minutes, or until the grain is tender.

5 Remove from the heat, drain any excess water and place the freekeh in a bowl.

6 Add the onion to the freekeh and stir well. Add in the garlic, paprika and chilli powder, along with the thyme, and mix well.

7 Spoon the mixture into the tomato halves, being careful not to split any of the skins so they continue to hold the mixture. Drizzle over a splash of olive oil and season with sea salt & pepper.

8 Return the stuffed tomatoes to the oven and cook for a further 10 – 12 minutes.

9 Place the fresh rocket leaves on a plate. Once cooked, place the tomatoes on the bed of rocket and top with a sprinkling of pine nuts to serve.

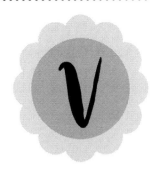

SERVES 2

ROASTED PEPPER & AUBERGINE COUSCOUS

Ingredients

- ½ aubergine, chopped
- 1 red pepper, chopped
- 1 yellow pepper, chopped
- 1 tbsp olive oil
- 1 clove of garlic, minced
- ½ tsp chilli powder

- A splash of vegan red wine
- A splash of red wine vinegar
- 1 tsp fresh basil, finely chopped
- A pinch of sea salt
- 100ml / 3½floz water
- 50g / 2oz couscous

- 1 tsp red lentils
- 1 tbsp Flaxseeds
- Fresh basil leaves to garnish

Method

1 Pre-heat the oven to 400F/200C /Gas 6.

2 Put the chopped aubergine & pepper into a bowl. Drizzle in the oil and add in the garlic and chilli powder, along with a splash of red wine and red wine vinegar.

3 Add in the chopped basil and sea salt then mix well. Spoon the mixture into a roasting dish and cook for 35 – 40 minutes, or until the vegetables are tender and beginning to crisp.

4 Meanwhile, bring the water to boil on a medium heat. Add in the couscous and lentils and allow to simmer for 10 minutes, or until cooked through and the water full absorbed. Drain off any excess water and place to one side.

5 Once cooked, remove the aubergine & pepper mixture from the oven and mix with the couscous and lentils, ready to serve.

6 Sprinkle over the flaxseeds and garnish with some fresh basil leaves.

CHEF'S NOTE
Add ½ red chilli, de-seeded to add a fiery kick to this delicious dinner.

NO-LAMB SHEPHERD'S PIE

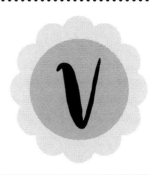

Ingredients

- 5 medium potatoes, peeled & chopped
- 1 tbsp olive oil
- 2 carrots, peeled & chopped
- ½ courgette, chopped
- ¼ onion, peeled & chopped
- 1 celery stick, chopped

- 50g/2oz mushrooms, chopped
- 1 clove of garlic, minced
- 150ml / 5floz vegetable stock
- Large splash of vegan red wine
- ¼ tsp tamarind paste
- Small pinch of cloves
- ½ tsp balsamic vinegar

- ½ tsp chilli powder
- 1 tbsp red lentils
- Sea salt & pepper
- 1 tbsp dairy-free spread
- 1 tbsp soya milk
- 1 tbsp grated vegan cheddar cheese

Method

1 Pre-heat the oven to 350F/180C /Gas 4.

2 Bring a pan of water to boil and add the chopped potatoes. Cook for 25 – 30 minutes, or until the potatoes are tender.

3 Meanwhile, warm the oil in a deep frying pan for 1 minute. Add into the frying pan the carrots, courgette, onion, celery, mushrooms and garlic and cook for 5 minutes until the vegetables begin to soften, stirring every minute or so.

4 Pour in the vegetable stock and add in the wine. Allow the mixture to simmer for 2 – 3 minutes. Then, add in the tamarind paste, cloves, vinegar, chilli powder and lentils, season with salt & pepper, and allow to simmer for a further 10 – 15 minutes. Remove from the heat and pour the mixture into a baking dish.

5 Once cooked, remove the potatoes from the heat, drain, and return them to the pan. Spoon in the dairy-free spread and mash the potatoes. Add in the soya milk, along with a seasoning of sea salt & pepper, and continue mashing until most of the lumps are gone.

6 Spoon the mashed potato over the vegetable mixture from the frying pan and smooth to completely cover the mixture, forming a potato top. Using a fork, gently press into the potato and lightly lift up, creating a rough pattern on top of the potato that will allow it to crisp slightly and add texture. Then, sprinkle on top the grated vegan cheese.

7 Place the baking dish on a baking tray, to catch any overspill just in case, and place in the oven for 30 – 35 minutes.

SERVES 2

ROASTED PUMPKIN AND CAULIFLOWER MEDLEY

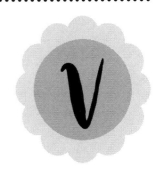

Ingredients

- 1 tbsp olive oil
- 200g/7oz pumpkin
- 50g/2oz butternut squash
- 100g/3½oz cauliflower
- ½ red pepper
- A large pinch of sea salt
- 1 tbsp olive oil

- 1 tsp fresh parsley, chopped
- A large pinch of sea salt
- A splash of fresh lemon juice
- A splash of vegan white wine vinegar
- A small pinch of turmeric
- 2 carrots, grated

- A handful of romaine lettuce leaves
- 1 tsp pomegranate seeds
- 1 tsp pumpkin seeds
- 1 tsp ground, roasted almonds

Method

1 Pre-heat the oven to 350F/180C /Gas 4.

2 Peel the pumpkin & squash, De-seed and chop the pumpkin, squash and pepper.

3 Splash the olive oil over the chopped pumpkin, butternut squash, cauliflower and red pepper, and season with the sea salt.

4 Cook in the oven for 20 – 25 minutes, or until tender and beginning to crisp.

5 Add into a bowl the extra olive oil, parsley, salt, lemon juice, white wine vinegar and turmeric. Mix well to create a dressing for the vegetables and place to one side ready to serve.

6 Arrange the romaine lettuce leaves on a plate to 'hold' the vegetables.

7 Once cooked, remove the vegetables from the oven and spoon onto the lettuce leaves.

8 Sprinkle on top the grated carrot and drizzle across the prepared dressing as desired. Top with seeds and almonds to serve.

CHEF'S NOTE

Pumpkin seeds are a good source of antioxidants, magnesium, zinc and fatty acids.

BUCKWHEAT STUFFED AUBERGINE

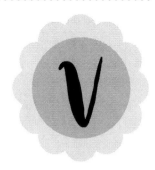

Ingredients

- 1 large aubergine, cut in half lengthways
- ½ large carrot, peeled & finely chopped
- 100g/3½oz raw buckwheat
- ¼ red onion, peeled & finely chopped
- 1 tsp tamari

- 1 tsp coriander
- ¼ red chilli, de-seeded & finely sliced
- 1 tsp pine nuts
- ½ tbsp olive oil
- Sea salt & pepper to season

Method

1 Pre-heat the oven to 350F/180C /Gas 4.

2 Take the halved aubergine and hollow out the main body. Chop some of the aubergine removed into dice-shaped chunks and place to one side.

3 Place the buckwheat in a pan and cover with water, allowing an extra centimetre of water above. Simmer on a medium heat for 15 – 20 minutes until tender. Stir occasionally and skim out any elements that float to the top.

4 Add the carrot and onion into a bowl, along with a small handful of the chopped aubergine. Add in the tamari, coriander, chilli and pine nuts and mix well. Drizzle in the oil, mix again and place the mixture to one side.

5 Once cooked, drain the buckwheat and rinse with warm water, before draining well again. Mix the cooked buckwheat with the aubergine and carrot mixture. Spoon the mixture into the aubergine skins and lightly brush the outside of the skin with any excess oil. Season with salt & pepper and roast in the oven for 35 – 40 minutes.

CHEF'S NOTE
Serve with tenderstem broccoli, or your choice of fresh, seasonal greens.

SWEET POTATO AND RED PEPPER FALAFEL

Ingredients

- 2 sweet potatoes, peeled & chopped
- 1 tsp olive oil
- 1 red pepper, de-seeded & finely chopped
- A large pinch of sea salt
- 400g/14oz tinned chickpeas, drained
- 2 tbsp plain flour

- 2 cloves of garlic, minced
- 1 tsp mild chilli powder
- 1 tsp ground cumin
- ½ tsp fresh coriander, finely chopped

Method

1 Pre-heat the oven to 400F/200C /Gas 6.

2 Place the sweet potato chunks on a baking tray and brush with the olive oil. Season with the sea salt and place in the oven for 25 minutes. Remove from the oven and add to the tray the chopped pepper.

3 Mix the pepper and sweet potatoes around the tray to coat the pepper in oil and turn the sweet potato to stop it from sticking. Return to the oven for another 15 – 20 minutes, or until tender.

4 Once cooked, remove from the oven and place in a bowl. Add in the chickpeas, flour and herbs and spices and mix well. Move the mixture into a food processor to blend the mixture together until a smooth, dough-like texture is formed.

5 Spoon out the mixture and roll each spoonful into a ball shape, no bigger than a golf ball. Place back on the baking tray, evenly spread out. Once you have used all of the mixture, place the tray in the oven and cook for 25 – 30 minutes, or until they are cooked through. Remove from the oven and serve.

CHEF'S NOTE

Low in saturated fat and very low in cholesterol and sodium, chickpeas contain high amounts of folate.

QUICK AND EASY CREAMY TOMATO PASTA

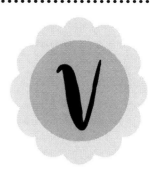

Ingredients

- 150g/5oz vegan fusilli pasta
- A small pinch of sea salt
- 200g/7oz passata
- ½ tsp ground paprika

- ½ tsp chilli powder
- 1 tbsp coconut cream
- Fresh basil leaves to garnish

Method

1 Bring a pan of water to boil with enough water in it to cover the pasta twice, at the least.

2 Add the pasta into the pan with a pinch of salt and boil for 10 – 12 minutes, or until the pasta is tender and cooked through.

3 Drain the pasta and then return it to the pan. Pour in the passata and stir well. Return the pan to the heat, but at a slightly reduced heat, and sprinkle in the spices, stirring well once more.

4 Allow to simmer for 1 – 2 minutes, stirring occasionally. Spoon in the coconut cream and mix well. Remove from the heat and serve.

5 Garnish with a fresh basil.

CHEF'S NOTE
Coconut flesh is highly nutritious and rich in fibre, vitamins C, E, B1, B3, B5 and B6 and minerals including iron, selenium, sodium, calcium, magnesium and phosphorous.

SPAGHETTI AND LENTIL BALLS

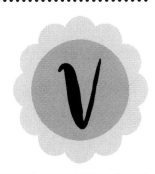

Ingredients

- 50g/2oz red lentils
- 50g/2oz green lentils
- 50g/2oz chickpeas, cooked
- ½ onion, peeled & chopped
- 2 cloves of garlic, minced
- 2 tbsp plain flour
- 2 tbsp hempseed oil

- ½ tsp fresh oregano, chopped
- 1 tsp fresh parsley, chopped
- ½ tsp fresh thyme, chopped
- 150g/5oz vegan spaghetti
- A pinch of sea salt
- 400g/14oz tinned chopped tomatoes

- 1 tbsp tomato puree
- 1 tsp ground paprika
- 1 tsp mild chilli powder
- ½ tsp dried mixed herbs
- Fresh basil to serve

Method

1 Pre-heat the oven to 400F/200C/Gas 6.

2 Cook and drain the lentils and chickpeas (or used tinned). Place the lentils, chickpeas and onion in a bowl and toss together. Add in the garlic, flour, oil and herbs & stir well.

3 Place into a food processor to blend the mixture together until a smooth, dough-like texture is formed.

4 Begin to spoon out the mixture and roll each spoonful into a ball shape, no bigger than a golf ball. Place back on a baking tray covered with grease-proof paper, evenly spaced out. Once you have used all of the mixture, place the tray in the oven and cook for 25 – 30 minutes, or until they are cooked through.

5 Meanwhile, bring a pan of water to boil and add in the spaghetti with a pinch of salt.

6 Boil the spaghetti for 10 – 12 minutes, or until cooked through, stirring occasionally to separate the strands and to prevent it from sticking to the bottom. While the spaghetti cooks, pour the tinned tomatoes into a saucepan with the tomato puree and spices and simmer on a low heat for 10 minutes, so that the mixture begins to thicken.

7 Once cooked, remove the spaghetti from the pan and drain before serving. Spoon the tomato mixture on top of the spaghetti and arrange the cooked lentil balls on top. Drizzle any remaining sauce lightly on top of the lentil balls and garnish with a fresh basil leaf to serve.

WINTER VEGETABLE BROTH

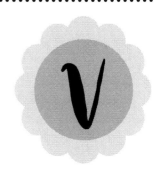

Ingredients

- 600ml/1 pint organic vegetable stock
- 1 potato, peeled & chopped
- 1 sweet potato, peeled & chopped
- ½ onion, peeled & chopped
- 1 large carrot, peeled & chopped
- ½ head cauliflower, chopped
- 1 celery stick, finely chopped
- 1 tbsp pearl barley
- 1 tsp red lentils
- A small pinch of curry powder
- Sea salt & pepper to season

Method

1 Bring the vegetable stock to boil in a saucepan and add in all of the vegetables.

2 Allow them to simmer for 10 minutes, stirring occasionally. Add in the pearl barley, red lentils, curry powder and season with salt & pepper.

3 Allow the mixture to simmer for a further 15 – 20 minutes, or until the vegetables are tender.

4 Once cooked through, remove from the head and gently mash the mixture a couple of times so that the vegetables are roughly broken up and simply serve.

CHEF'S NOTE
Barley is high in fibre and can help improve digestion.

ROASTED SWEET POTATO AND AUBERGINE CURRY

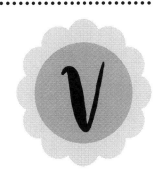

Ingredients

- 1 sweet potato, chopped
- ½ aubergine, chopped
- 1 tsp olive oil
- A pinch of sea salt
- 1 tsp coconut oil
- ½ red onion, chopped
- 1 large clove of garlic, minced

- 1 small red chilli, de-seeded & finely sliced
- ½ tbsp tomato puree
- A pinch of fresh root ginger, grated
- ½ tsp fresh coriander, finely chopped

- ½ tsp ground paprika
- ¾ tsp garam masala
- 250g/9oz tinned chopped tomatoes
- 100g/3½oz brown rice
- 1 tbsp coconut cream
- Fresh coriander to garnish

Method

1 Pre-heat the oven to 400F/200C /Gas 6.

2 Toss the sweet potato chunks and aubergine in the olive oil and place on a baking tray. Season with sea salt and place in the oven for 35 – 40 minutes, or until the vegetables are tender and beginning to crisp.

3 Heat the coconut oil in a pan on a medium heat and add the red onion, garlic and chilli. Cook for 2–3 minutes so they start to soften, stirring regularly.

4 Add in the tomato puree and the herbs and spices and stir well, allowing to cook for another couple of minutes.

5 Add in the tinned tomatoes, stir well, and allow the mixture to simmer for 5 minutes or until it begins to thicken.

6 Once cooked, remove the sweet potato and aubergine from the oven and add to the tomato mixture in the pan, stirring well. Reduce to a low heat, cover, and allow the curry to simmer for 45 minutes, stirring occasionally.

7 Bring a pan of water to boil and cook the brown rice until tender. Once cooked, drain and serve the rice, and spoon on top the curry mixture ready to serve.

8 Drizzle over the coconut cream and garnish with some fresh coriander.

HUMMUS CRUSTED MUSHROOM

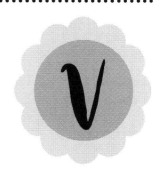

Ingredients

- 150g/5oz chickpeas, cooked & drained
- ½ clove of garlic, minced
- 2 tsp tahini paste
- 25ml/1floz vegetable stock
- 2 tsp olive oil
- 1 tbsp freshly squeezed lemon juice
- A pinch of sea salt & pepper
- 2 large Portobello mushrooms, stalks removed
- A splash of olive oil

Method

1 Pre-heat the oven to 325F/170C /Gas 3.

2 To make the hummus, simply blend together the chickpeas, garlic, tahini paste, stock, oil and lemon juice.

3 Add in sea salt & pepper to season, blend once more and place to one side.

4 Spoon the hummus over the mushrooms and spread to cover most of its surface. Cook for 20 – 25 minutes, or until the hummus crust turns golden and starts to crisp and the mushroom is tender.

CHEF'S NOTE
Mushrooms are high in antioxidants, selenium, and vitamin D.

SERVES 2

SLOW-COOKED SAUSAGE AND MIXED BEAN CHILLI

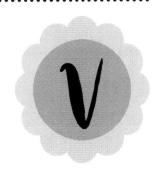

Ingredients

- 1 tsp olive oil
- ½ onion, peeled & chopped
- ½ yellow pepper, de-seeded & chopped
- ½ clove of garlic, minced
- 2 vegan sausages,
- 50ml/2floz vegetable stock
- 200g/7oz tinned tomatoes

- 1 tsp chilli powder
- 1 tsp paprika
- A small pinch of granulated coffee
- 50g/2oz red kidney beans, cooked & drained
- 25g/1oz lima beans, cooked & drained
- 50g/2oz black beans, cooked & drained

Method

1 Pre-heat the oven to 300F/150C /Gas 2 or switch the slow cooker on low.

2 Warm the oil in a pan and add in the onion, pepper and garlic. Cook for a couple of minutes and then add in the vegan sausages.

3 Cook for a further 5 minutes, stirring and turning the sausages, until the vegetables have softened and the sausages sealed. Remove the pan from the heat and place to one side. Remove the sausages and cut into chunky slices.

4 Add the vegetable stock, tinned tomatoes, spices and coffee into a casserole dish, along with the onion & pepper mixture from the pan and the chopped sausages.

5 Stir the mixture well and then add in the mixed beans. Cover and cook in the oven for 3 – 4 hours, removing the lid or cover for the final 20 minutes. If using a slow cooker, allow to cook for 5 – 6 hours. Simply serve from the dish.

CHEF'S NOTE
The vitamin B6 in paprika promotes good eye health.

CREAMY QUINOA RISOTTO

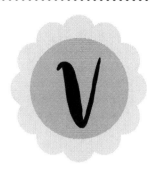

Ingredients

- 1 tsp olive oil
- 1 carrot, peeled & chopped
- 1 celery stick, finely chopped
- 1 Litre/3 pints water
- A pinch of sea salt

- 150g/5oz quinoa, rinsed
- ½ tsp nutmeg
- 1 tbsp soya cream
- Fresh coriander to serve

Method

1 Warm the olive oil in a pan and add in the carrot and celery.

2 Cook for 4–5 minutes, until the carrot and celery are softening slightly.

3 Remove from the heat and place to one side. Bring the water to boil in a saucepan. Add in a pinch of salt with the quinoa and carrot and celery from the pan and simmer for 10 minutes, stirring continuously.

4 Sprinkle in the nutmeg and allow to simmer for a further 5 minutes, or until the quinoa is fully cooked and expanded.

5 When cooked, drain any excess water and mix in the soya cream, allowing the quinoa mixture to warm it through before serving.

6 Garnish with fresh coriander and serve.

CHEF'S NOTE
With a subtle, creamy taste soya cream has almost half the fat of non-vegan single cream.

GREEN PEPPER FALAFEL BURGER

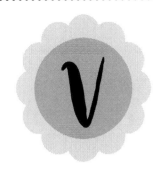

Ingredients

- 1 tsp olive oil
- ½ green pepper, de-seeded & finely chopped
- A large pinch of sea salt
- 400g/14oz tinned chickpeas, cooked & drained
- 2 tbsp plain flour
- 2 cloves of garlic, minced
- ½ tsp fresh coriander, finely chopped
- 1 tsp ground cumin
- ½ tsp fresh parsley, finely chopped
- 4 romaine lettuce leaves
- 1 large tomato, sliced
- 1 tsp of your preferred vegan sauce (mayonnaise, ketchup, etc.)

Method

1 Pre-heat the oven to 400F/200C/Gas 6 and line a baking tray with grease-proof paper.

2 Meanwhile, warm the oil in a pan and add in the chopped pepper, seasoning with salt. Cook for 3–4 minutes, until the pepper is beginning to soften. Once cooked, remove from the pan and place in a food processor, or bowl if using a hand blender.

3 Add in the chickpeas and flour, herbs and spices and blend the mixture together until a smooth, dough-like texture is formed.

4 Spoon out the mixture and separate into two large balls. Place on the baking tray and gently flatten the mixture so it spreads, evenly, into a burger-like shape.

5 Ensure they are well-spaced apart and then cook in the oven for 20–25 minutes, or until they are golden and crisp. Once cooked, remove from the oven and serve warm.

6 Use the romaine lettuce leaves as a 'bun', placing the falafel burger and some tomato slices between the leaves. Add a small spoonful of your choice of vegan sauce and serve.

CHEF'S NOTE

Chickpeas are high in fibre and protein, and contain several key vitamins and minerals.

HALLOUMI PESTO PASTA

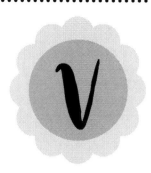

Ingredients

- 3 tbsp hempseed oil
- 1 large bunch of fresh basil, finely chopped
- ½ clove of garlic, minced
- 3 tbsp pine nuts
- ½ tsp freshly squeezed lemon juice
- A pinch of sea salt
- 150g/5oz vegan fusilli pasta
- 200g/7oz vegan halloumi, chopped

Method

1 To make the pesto pasta sauce, simply add all of the ingredients either into a food processor and blend until smooth. Place in a bowl to one side ready to use.

2 Bring a pan of water to boil and add in the pasta, with a pinch of salt, and boil for 10 – 12 minutes, or until cooked through.

3 Meanwhile, warm a frying pan on a medium heat to cook the halloumi. Add the halloumi into the pan and cook for 2 – 3 minutes on each side, or until golden.

4 Once cooked, drain the pasta and return to the pan on a low heat. Spoon in the pesto pasta sauce and warm through, stirring the pasta continuously.

5 Either add the chopped halloumi in and stir once more before serving or arrange on top of the pasta to serve.

CHEF'S NOTE
Ensure you choose vegan tofu halloumi not regular goats cheese halloumi.

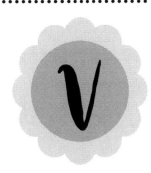

MINT AND GARLIC BUTTER GREENS

SERVES 1

Ingredients

- 1 tbsp almond butter
- 1 clove of garlic, minced
- A pinch of sea salt
- A pinch of dried mixed herbs
- A large pinch of mint, freshly chopped
- 8 stalks of tenderstem broccoli

- 50g/2oz green beans, chopped
- 25g/1oz broad beans
- 50g/2oz asparagus spears
- 1 tsp pine nuts
- 1 tsp peanuts, chopped
- Sea salt & pepper to season

Method

1 Pre-heat the oven to 350F/180C /Gas 4.

2 In a small bowl, mix together the almond butter, garlic, sea salt, herb and mint until it is smoothly combined and place to one side ready to use later.

3 Bring a large saucepan of water to boil. Add in the broccoli, green beans, broad beans and asparagus and boil for 7 - 10 minutes. The greens should be turning tender, but not completely cooked through just yet.

4 Drain and place in a roasting dish. Spoon over the garlic and mint butter and gently mix the greens around so they are evenly covered in the butter as it melts.

5 Sprinkle on top the nuts and season generously with sea salt & pepper. Roast in the oven for 10 – 15 minutes and serve.

CHEF'S NOTE

Broccoli is great for heart health as it contains fibre, fatty acids and vitamins that help regulate blood pressure in the body.

SERVES 2

CARROT AND RED PEPPER BURGUNDY

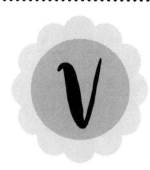

Ingredients

- ½ tbsp dairy-free spread
- 2 carrots, peeled & chopped
- 1 red pepper, de-seeded & chopped
- ½ onion, peeled & chopped
- 1 clove of garlic, minced
- 75g/3oz button mushrooms, halved
- 150ml/5floz vegetable stock
- 200ml/7floz vegan red wine
- 6 shallots, peeled and halved
- 1 ½ tbsp plain flour
- 1 bay leaf
- 1 tsp fresh thyme, finely chopped
- A pinch of fresh coriander, finely chopped
- Sea salt & pepper to season

Method

1 Melt the dairy-free spread in the pan on a medium heat.

2 Add into the pan the carrots, red pepper and onion. Sauté for 3 – 4 minutes, stirring occasionally.

3 Add in the garlic and mushrooms and sauté for a further 2 – 3 minutes, allowing the vegetables to soften.

4 Bring the vegetable stock to a boil and add in the vegetables from the pan, stirring well. Pour in the red wine, add the shallots and allow to simmer for 5 minutes on a low heat.

5 Sieve in the flour, add in the herbs and season generously with sea salt & pepper. Allow the mixture to simmer for 45 minutes on a low heat.

6 Once the vegetables are tender, remove from the heat and serve.

CHEF'S NOTE
Not all wine is vegan so choose carefully taking note of the how the wine is clarified.

VEGETABLE BOLOGNESE

Ingredients

- 1 tsp olive oil
- ½ onion, peeled & chopped
- 2 carrots, peeled & finely chopped
- 1 red pepper, de-seeded & finely chopped
- 1 courgette & 1 stick celery, chopped
- 6 mushrooms, finely chopped
- 1 clove of garlic, minced

- 150ml/5floz vegetable stock
- 400g/14oz tinned tomatoes, chopped
- A splash of vegan red wine
- 1 tbsp tomato puree
- ½ tsp each sugar & mixed herbs & paprika
- 150g/5oz vegan spaghetti
- 1 tsp vegan style Parmesan cheese

Method

1 Heat the oil in a saucepan and add in all of the vegetables and garlic.

2 Cook the vegetables on a medium heat for 5 - 7 minutes, stirring occasionally. Once the vegetables have begun to soften add in the vegetable stock and simmer for 5 minutes.

3 Add in the tinned tomatoes, red wine, tomato puree, sugar, mixed herbs and paprika and simmer for a further 15 - 20 minutes, or until the vegetables are cooked through.

4 Meanwhile, bring a separate saucepan of water to boil and add the spaghetti in. Boil for 10 – 12 minutes, until the spaghetti is cooked through. Once cooked, drain the spaghetti and serve.

5 Spoon the bolognese mixture on top of the spaghetti and serve with a sprinkling of the vegan Parmesan cheese.

CHEF'S NOTE
Unrefined sugar is sometimes referred to as raw sugar.

WHITE STEW AND DUMPLINGS

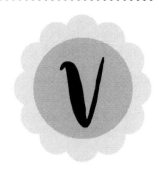

Ingredients

- 25g/1oz dairy-free spread
- 75g/3oz self-raising flour
- 25ml/1floz soya milk
- 25ml/1floz pureed silken tofu
- A pinch of salt & pepper
- A small pinch of mixed herbs
- 1 tbsp olive oil

- ½ onion, peeled & chopped
- ½ clove of garlic, minced
- 1 celery stick, chopped
- 1 small potato, peeled & chopped
- ½ turnip, peeled & chopped
- ½ parsnip, peeled & chopped

- 250ml/8½floz boiling vegetable stock
- 50ml/2floz dry vegan white wine
- Sea salt & pepper
- 1 tbsp pearl barley

Method

1 Pre-heat the oven to 350F/180C /Gas 4.

2 In a bowl, use your fingers to rub together the spread and flour to combine the ingredients into a crumble-style mixture.

3 Add in the soya milk and silken tofu and repeat the process. Season with salt & pepper and add in the mixed herbs. Continue to rub and mix until a dough-like texture is created.

4 Add a splash more milk if needed. Roll the dumpling mixture into balls, similar in size to a golf ball, and place to one side.

5 Heat the oil in a pan and add in all of the vegetables and garlic. Cook the vegetables on a medium heat for 4 – 5 minutes, stirring occasionally, until the edges begin to soften and look golden.

6 Remove from the heat and place into a casserole dish, pouring the vegetable stock on top. Add in the wine, season, and stir well. Sprinkle in the pearl barley and stir the stew once more before adding in the prepared dumplings.

7 Put a lid on the dish, or cover with foil, and cook in the oven for 45 minutes. Then, remove the lid or foil and return to the oven for 10 – 15 minutes, or until the dumplings begin to crisp. Remove from the oven and serve.

Skinny
VEGAN
Desserts

MELT IN THE MIDDLE MINI CHOCOLATE PUDDINGS

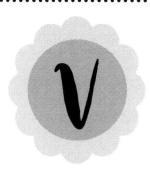

Ingredients

- 50g/2oz cocoa butter
- 50g/2oz dark vegan chocolate
- 75g/3oz soft brown sugar
- 1½ tsp baking soda

- 1½ tbsp white vinegar
- A dash of vanilla extract
- 25g/1oz plain flour

Method

1 Pre-heat the oven to 400F/200C /Gas 6.

2 Butter two ramekin dishes well. Bring a small saucepan of water to simmer. Place the cocoa butter and dark chocolate in an oven-proof bowl and place on top of the saucepan, ensuring that the bottom of the bowl does not touch the water.

3 Allow the chocolate and butter to melt into a mixture, gently stirring. Then add in the sugar and stir well.

4 In a separate bowl, mix together the white vinegar and baking soda until completely combined.

5 Remove the bowl of chocolate mixture from the heat and add the vinegar and baking soda mixture in, stirring well.

6 Add in the vanilla extract and sieve in the flour. Stir the mixture well and then pour into the ramekin dishes. Cook in the oven for 12 – 15 minutes, until the tops are soft to touch.

7 Once cooked, remove from the oven and allow to rest for 10 minutes. Using a knife, gently insert it around the edge of the pudding to softly separate it from the ramekin dish. Place a plate for serving on top of the ramekin dish, and flip over. Remove the ramekin dish and serve.

CHEF'S NOTE
Serve with a dollop of vegan ice cream.

VERY BERRY YOGHURT

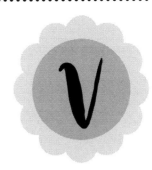

Ingredients

- 175ml/6floz vegan yoghurt
- 1 tsp agave nectar
- 25g/1oz blueberries
- 25g/1oz blackberries
- 25g/1oz raspberries
- 25g/1oz redcurrants
- 1 tsp desiccated coconut
- 1 tsp chia seeds

Method

1 Mix the yoghurt and agave nectar together and place to one side.

2 Simply toss the berries and currants together in a bowl and lightly mash a few times.

3 Spoon the yoghurt onto a plate or into a bowl to serve and top with the berry mixture.

4 Sprinkle on top the desiccated coconut and chia seeds to serve.

CHEF'S NOTE

Berries are packed with antioxidants and help to keep skin clear. For ease, you can make this using frozen fruit also.

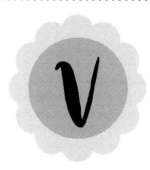

APPLE AND RHUBARB CRUMBLE

SERVES 2

Ingredients

- 3 large cooking apples, peeled & chopped
- A handful of fresh rhubarb, washed & finely chopped
- 1 tsp light brown sugar
- ½ tsp ground cinnamon
- 75g/3oz plain flour
- 50g/2oz almond butter
- ½ tbsp demerara sugar

Method

1 Pre-heat the oven to 350F/180C /Gas 4.

2 Place the chopped apples and rhubarb in a small baking dish and sprinkle in the sugar and cinnamon, mixing the ingredients together well.

3 In a separate bowl, add the plain flour, almond butter and sugar and stir.

4 Using your hands, rub the mixture together, crumbling the pieces, until a crumble like texture and mixture is achieved.

5 Sprinkle the crumble mixture on top of the apple and rhubarb until it is evenly covered. Bake in the oven for 35 – 40 minutes, or until the crumble is golden and the fruit softened.

CHEF'S NOTE
Top with your preferred choice of crushed or ground nuts for nuttier flavour.

SUMMER FRUIT SALAD

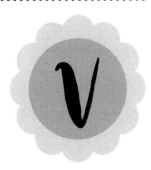

Ingredients

- 50g/2oz strawberries, chopped
- 25g/1oz raspberries, chopped
- A pinch of unrefined sugar
- 50g/2oz watermelon, peeled chopped
- 50g/2oz mango, peeled & chopped
- 50g/2oz pineapple, peeled & chopped
- 1 tsp desiccated coconut

Method

1 Place the strawberries and raspberries in a bowl and mash together well.

2 Add in a pinch of sugar and stir again. Using a hand blender, blend until a smooth, liquid-like mixture is formed and place to one side.

3 Simply toss the watermelon, mango and pineapple in a bowl, ready to serve.

4 Drizzle on top the strawberry and raspberry sauce and top with a sprinkling of desiccated coconut.

CHEF'S NOTE

For a warming contrast, sauté the strawberries and raspberries to create a warm, gooey sauce to drizzle on top.

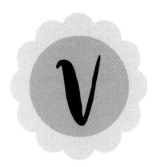

COLD CHOCOLATE AND COCONUT PUDDING

SERVES 2

Ingredients

- 150ml/5floz coconut milk
- 60ml/2floz coconut cream
- ½ tbsp maple syrup
- A dash of vanilla extract
- ½ tsp flaxseeds
- 25g/1oz dark vegan chocolate, grated
- A pinch of desiccated coconut

Method

1 Pour the coconut milk, cream, maple syrup, vanilla extract and flaxseeds into a food processor and blend until a smooth mixture is created.

2 Add in the grated chocolate and stir well. Pour the mixture into two ramekin dishes.

3 Place in the fridge and leave to cool for 2 hours. Remove from the fridge and sprinkle on top the desiccated coconut and any leftover grated chocolate.

4 Return to the fridge for a further 2–3 hours, or longer if you can to allow the mixture to set.

5 Once set, remove from the fridge and serve straight away.

CHEF'S NOTE
For best results, allow the mixture to set in the fridge overnight.

KIWI MOJITO SLUSH

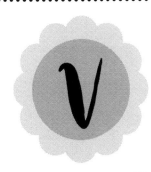

Ingredients

- The juice of ½ a lime, freshly squeezed
- 1 tsp fresh mint, finely chopped
- ½ kiwi, peeled & finely chopped
- A pinch of light brown sugar
- 25ml/1floz white rum
- 50ml/2floz soda water
- A handful of crushed ice
- Lime peel to garnish
- Fresh mint leaf to garnish

Method

1 Put the lime juice, mint, kiwi, sugar, soda water and rum into a food processor, or a bowl if using a hand blender, and blend into a smooth mixture.

2 Place the crushed ice into a glass, or bowl, ready to serve, and pour over the lime and mint mixture, allowing it to filter through the crushed ice.

3 Garnish with a twisted piece of fresh lime peel and a mint leaf to serve.

CHEF'S NOTE

Virtually all spirits —bourbon, whiskey, vodka, gin, and rum—are vegan. Nearly all distilled spirits are vegan except for cream-based liqueurs and products that mention honey on the label.

CHERRY MUFFINS

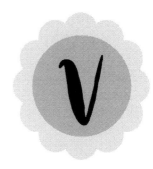

Ingredients

- 50g/2oz caster sugar
- 1 tbsp almond butter
- 100ml/3½floz soya milk
- 125g/4oz plain flour

- 1 ½ tsp baking soda
- A small pinch of salt
- 1 tsp desiccated coconut
- 40g/1½oz glacier cherries, chopped

Method

1 Pre-heat the oven to 350F/180C /Gas 4.

2 In a bowl, combine the sugar and almond butter. Pour in some of the soya milk and stir well until a smooth mixture is achieved.

3 Gradually add the rest of the milk, stirring continuously. Sieve in the flour and baking soda and mix well. Add in a pinch of salt, the coconut and cherries and stir well once more.

4 Spoon the mixture into muffin cases and bake in the oven for 15 – 20 minutes, or until cooked through.

5 To check, pierce a knife into the middle of one cake; if when withdrawn it is clear, they are cooked, if some mixture is present, they may need a few minutes longer.

CHEF'S NOTE
These are delicious served warm or can be cooled and saved for a sweet breakfast treat.

WHITE CHOCOLATE AND RASPBERRY CAKE LOAF

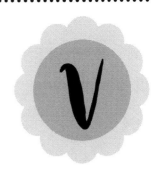

Ingredients

- 100g/3½oz caster sugar
- 2 tbsp cocoa butter
- 1 tbsp almond butter
- 200ml /7floz almond milk
- 225g / 8oz plain flour
- 3 tsp baking soda
- ½ tsp crushed pecan nuts
- A dash of vanilla extract
- 40g/1½oz vegan white chocolate
- 25g/1oz raspberries, chopped
- 1 tbsp freshly whipped dairy-free cream
- A small handful of whole raspberries to serve

Method

1 Pre-heat the oven to 350F/180C /Gas 4.

2 Butter a loaf tin well, or line with grease-proof paper. In a bowl, combine the sugar, cocoa butter and almond butter.

3 Pour in half of the almond milk and stir well until a smooth mixture is achieved. Gradually add the rest of the milk, stirring continuously.

4 Sieve in the flour and baking soda and mix well. Add in the pecan nuts, vanilla extract, chocolate and raspberries and stir well once more.

5 Spoon the mixture into the loaf tin or dish and bake in the oven for 30 – 35 minutes, or until cooked through.

6 Remove from the oven and allow to cool for 10 – 15 minutes. Use a teaspoon to decorate the cake with spots of cream and top each 'spot' with raspberries to serve.

CHEF'S NOTE

Pecans are excellent sources of manganese and copper, two minerals that boost overall metabolic health.

SWEET ROASTED PEAR

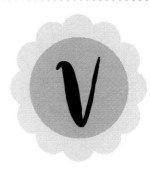

Ingredients

- 2 pears, cored and halved
- 2 tbsp oats
- 1 tbsp maple syrup

- A pinch of cinnamon
- A small pinch of nutmeg
- 1 tsp pecan nuts, ground

Method

1 Pre-heat the oven to 325F/170C /Gas 3.

2 Gently spoon about ½ the pear from each pear half, finely chop it and place in a bowl. Add in the oats, maple syrup and spices and stir well.

3 Spoon the mixture back into the pear halves and cover slightly. Use any excess maple syrup to coat the pear skins.

4 Roast in the oven for 20 – 25 minutes, until golden and tender. Sprinkle on top the pecan nuts to serve.

CHEF'S NOTE

Oats are among the healthiest grains on earth. They're a gluten-free whole grain and a great source of important vitamins, minerals, fibre and antioxidants.

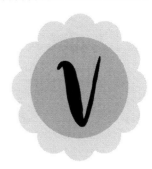

SERVES 8

PEANUT BUTTER AND JELLY COOKIES

Ingredients

- 75g/3oz almond butter
- 40g/1½oz vegan peanut butter
- 50g/2oz brown caster sugar
- 3 tbsp maple syrup
- 125g/4oz plain flour
- 1 tbsp peanuts, chopped
- 1 tbsp glacier cherries, finely chopped

Method

1 Pre-heat the oven to 350F/180C /Gas 4 and line a baking tray with grease-proof paper.

2 In a bowl, combine almond butter, peanut butter and sugar. Stir in the maple syrup and sieve in half of the flour. Mix well, and gradually add in the remaining flour, stirring continuously.

3 Add in the chopped peanuts and cherries and stir well. Scoop out the mixture to form 8 large spoonfuls on the baking tray, well-spaced out.

4 Gently press down on the mixture and mould a cookie shape ready for baking. Bake for 10 – 15 minutes.

5 Allow the cookies to cool for 5 minutes before serving.

CHEF'S NOTE

For a gooey centre, mould the mixture so it is less wide but thicker before placing in the oven and bake for just 10 minutes.

VODKA WINTER BERRY CHILLED COMPOTE

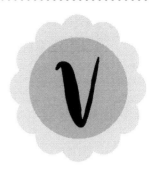

Ingredients

- 1 tsp almond butter
- 50g/2oz blackberries
- 25g/1oz blackcurrants
- 25g/1oz raspberries
- ½ tsp brown sugar
- 25ml/1floz vodka
- 75ml/3floz vegan yoghurt

- 75g/3floz vegan cream
- ½ tsp maple syrup
- 50g/2oz vegan granola
- 4 crushed vegan biscuits of choice (as close to a Digestive style biscuit as possible)
- Raspberries to garnish

Method

1 Melt the almond butter in a small pan on a low heat.

2 Mash the berries together in a bowl, along with the sugar. Add the berry mixture to the pan and simmer for 1 minute. Then, add in the vodka and simmer for a further 3 – 4 mins, stirring continuously until a coulis style mixture is created. Remove from the heat and place to one side.

3 Pour the yoghurt and cream into a bowl, stir in the maple syrup and place to one side.

4 Mix the granola and crushed biscuits together and spoon them into 2 ramekin dishes to create a base.

5 Pack it down tightly with a spoon so the mixture is compact. Spoon on top the yoghurt and cream and level it out with a spoon.

6 Drizzle the berry mixture from the pan on top and place in the fridge for 2 – 3 hours, or longer if you can.

7 Remove from the fridge and garnish with a raspberry to serve.

CHEF'S NOTE

These can easily be prepared the night before and kept in the fridge until serving.

DARK RUM & CHOCOLATE FAKE CHEESECAKE

Ingredients

- 25g/1oz cocoa butter
- 25g/1oz dark vegan chocolate
- 75ml/3floz vegan yoghurt
- 75ml/3floz vegan cream
- 1 tbsp cocoa powder
- 25ml/1floz dark rum
- 1 tsp pecan nuts, crushed

Method

1 Bring a small saucepan of water to simmer.

2 Place the cocoa butter and dark chocolate in an oven-proof bowl and place on top of the saucepan, ensuring that the bottom of the bowl does not touch the water. Allow the chocolate and butter to melt into a mixture, gently stirring.

3 In a separate bowl, mix together the yoghurt, cream, cocoa powder and rum.

4 Pour the mixture into 2 ramekin dishes and level the mixture with the back of a spoon. Then, gently drizzle on top the melted chocolate mixture, covering the yoghurt entirely.

5 Sprinkle on top the crushed pecan nuts and place in the fridge for 3 – 4 hours for the chocolate to set.

6 Once set, remove from the fridge and serve.

CHEF'S NOTE

Simply exclude the rum for an alcohol-free version, or swap with your preferred spirit of choice.

BLUEBERRY RICE PUDDING

········ *Ingredients* ·········

- 1 litre/1½ pints almond milk
- 50g/2oz arborio rice, rinsed
- 40g/1 ½oz caster sugar
- A small pinch of nutmeg
- 1 tbsp vanilla essence

- 50g/2oz blueberries
- ½ tsp maple syrup
- 1 tsp crushed almonds
- 1 tsp pomegranate seeds

········ *Method* ·········

1 Pre-heat the oven to 325F/170C /Gas 3.

2 Bring a small saucepan of water to simmer. In a saucepan warm through the almond milk on a low heat, and gradually increase the heat to bring the milk to a simmer.

3 Add in the rice, sugar, nutmeg and vanilla essence and stir well. Allow the mixture to simmer for 25 – 30 minutes, stirring every few minutes to ensure the rice does not gather and stick to the bottom of the pan. A thick, gloopy mixture should evenly form. Once achieved, remove from the pan and spoon the rice pudding into a small oven-proof dish, or split across 2 ramekin dishes. Place in the oven to cook for 20 – 25 minutes.

4 Place the blueberries in a bowl with the maple syrup and crushed almonds.

5 Mash the mixture together ready to serve. Remove the rice pudding from the oven and allow 5 minutes to cool.

6 Spoon on top the blueberry mixture and sprinkle on top pomegranate seeds to serve.

CHEF'S NOTE
Pomegranates are rich in vitamin C, potassium, and fibre.

Printed in Great Britain
by Amazon